CW01212943

PRESCRIPTION: ICE CREAM

PRESCRIPTION: ICE CREAM

A Doctor's Journey to Discover What Matters

ALASTAIR MCALPINE

MACMILLAN

First published in 2024
by Pan Macmillan South Africa
Private Bag X19
Northlands
Johannesburg
2116
www.panmacmillan.co.za

ISBN 978-1-77010-804-2
e-ISBN 978-1-77010-805-9

© 2024 Alastair McAlpine

All rights reserved. No part of this publication may be reproduced, stored in or introduced into a retrieval system, or transmitted, in any form or by any means (electronic, mechanical, photocopying, recording or otherwise), without the prior written permission of the publisher. Any person who does any unauthorised act in relation to this publication may be liable to criminal prosecution and civil claims for damages.

Editing by Jane Bowman
Proofreading by Sean Fraser
Design and typesetting by Nyx Design
Cover design by mr design

Printed by novus print, a division of Novus Holdings

Dedicated to:
Roy and Helen (my past)
Laura (my present)
Grayson (my future)

'That message is simple: When you come to one of the many moments in life when you must give an account of yourself, provide a ledger of what you have been, and done, and meant to the world, do not, I pray, discount that you filled a dying man's days with a sated joy.'
– Paul Kalanithi, *When Breath Becomes Air*

'The truth is, you should consider yourself lucky if you even occasionally get to make someone – anyone – feel a little better.'
– John 'J.D.' Dorian, *Scrubs*

Contents

A Note on the Text ... xi

PART 1: The Presentation
Chapter 1   The Firm ... 3
Chapter 2   A Nursery of Interns ... 35
Chapter 3   Certified ... 53
Chapter 4   On the Clock ... 73
Chapter 5   Comrades ... 86
Chapter 6   The Pit ... 99
Chapter 7   Active Labour ... 125
Chapter 8   Brothers in Arms ... 141

PART 2: The History
Chapter 9   Powerless ... 155
Chapter 10   Take Two ... 184
Chapter 11   Sipho and the Beetroot ... 216

PART 3: The Prescription
Chapter 12   Witnessing Jason's Journey ... 257
Chapter 13   PaedsPal ... 269
Chapter 14   What Makes You Happy? ... 283
Chapter 15   The Healing Properties of Ice Cream ... 293

Reflections on Going Viral ... 301
Acknowledgements ... 309

A Note on the Text

In order to respect and preserve the privacy of patients, doctors, colleagues, friends and those struggling with addiction, in writing this memoir I have changed various details, such as names and key identifiers, while maintaining the relevant facts.

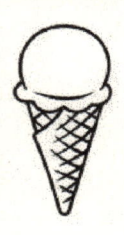

PART 1
The Presentation

Chapter 1
THE FIRM

At 10:30pm, when ward 30 explodes, I think back to the tranquility of the morning. The morning is when the Chris Hani Baragwanath Hospital in Soweto is at its most peaceful.

That day – my first at the hospital – had started just over fifteen hours earlier, after a night of restless sleep. In the darkness, I kept glancing over at the new lanyard dangling from the nearby chair, squinting to see if the word 'Doctor' was still on the name badge, and hadn't been erased after some higher power realised that a mistake had been made; that I couldn't possibly be ready to start treating actual patients on my own. A persistent nausea had settled deep in my abdomen, replacing the excitement that had been present since graduation two months earlier. I tried to calm my thudding heart and reminded myself that six years of medical school had prepared me for this; I was ready. But no sooner had my breathing settled than doubts began seeping into my brain like black ink through water. What if someone had an illness I had never studied? If there was an emergency would I remember what to do? What if I made a mistake and someone suffered or died as a result?

PART 1: THE PRESENTATION

This gnawing anxiety was compounded by the reputation of what was to be my workplace for the next two years. Baragwanath, or Bara (as it was generally referred to) was infamous. Stories had filtered all the way back to Cape Town that it regularly reduced junior doctors to tears. It was a hospital that could shatter you if you weren't able to handle the pressure. Those who had survived their internship at Baragwanath wore it like a badge of honour and had the grizzled, slightly damaged look of war veterans who had 'seen things', rather than junior professionals with a two-year medical apprenticeship under their belts.

When the shrill of the alarm clock pierced the quiet morning, I was so wired I almost jumped out of bed. To calm my thudding pulse, I rechecked my medical bag for what felt like the twentieth time since the night before. Stethoscope? Lying like a snake poised and ready to strike. Folder for documents and ward lists? Propped up proudly on the side of the bag. Well-thumbed *Internal Medicine* handbook from med school? Bookmarked and ready to be surreptitiously checked between patients. I glanced at the white coat hanging in my cupboard and was relieved that this piece of attire was not required at Baragwanath. I had always found wearing it stuffy and unnecessary; an extra piece of clothing in a withering climate that quickly reduced the crispest of extraneous layers to limp, damp cloth. With the sun gently rising, I grabbed a cup of coffee and a piece of toast and headed to the hospital.

Easing down the harsh concrete highway, I noticed on the horizon a gentle plume of smoke rising from the informal settlements and modest houses that surround Baragwanath. This haze signified an entire populace getting ready for the day. A thousand breakfasts being prepared, old bones and joints creaking to life, fresh-faced children being roughly washed and readied for school in crisp uniforms. Above lay the extraordinary blue of the African sky. Perhaps it was my adrenaline pumping, perhaps it was my senses on a state of high alert, but it was a startling sight this particular morning. On a sunny day, it is bluer and deeper than any ocean, and I found myself staring at it as I nervously shifted gear while waiting at a traffic light.

The moment of serenity was shattered by a high-pitched horn from an impatient minibus taxi behind me, upset that I had not pulled off the millisecond the light turned green. With a vaguely dismissive gesture from his window, more out of a sense of obligation than real anger, the taxi driver zoomed around me and sped off to collect his next cargo of passengers.

The drive to Soweto from the leafy, middle-class suburbs of Johannesburg was a surreal experience; a real-time journey through the glaring disparities of wealth that exist in South Africa. The tree-lined streets in front of enormous, high-walled houses quickly gave way to more modest, single-storeyed homes before the ubiquitous mine dumps that pock the outskirts of the city indicate you have reached the edge of where apartheid's planners intended white people to live. Beyond this, everything becomes a lot more haphazard, and on the southern border, the cruelly – and ironically – named 'Golden Highway' takes you to Klipfontein Road, one of the arteries that feeds the sprawling area of Soweto.

Soweto is not an informal settlement in the traditional sense of the phrase. Apartheid's architects wanted black South Africans to be far enough away from white South Africans to prevent unnecessary mingling, but close enough that their precious labour could power the goldmines that were springing up like pustules on the semi-arid landscape. Despite a crippling lack of resources, infrastructure, or support, it has, despite the incredible odds against it, thrived.

PART 1: THE PRESENTATION

Mostly due to the ingenuity and resilience of its inhabitants.

New York may be the city that never sleeps but Soweto is the town that never stops hustling. From well before the sun rises, to long after it has set, there is a relentless electricity and energy to the place. Taxi horns are constantly blown, people chatter and wave, wares are set out beside the road, and haggling and bartering is exchanged rapid-fire between inhabitants. Driving down the road, I saw a man selling a local delicacy: the legs and beaks of a chicken, colloquially referred to as a 'walkie talkie'.

I was glad that I had done a practice run the day before because the massive area of Soweto is poorly signposted and easy to get lost in. During its history, the township grew and expanded organically and haphazardly, rather than through any foresight by experienced planners. It reminded me, in some ways, of the anatomy of the chest; evolving slowly in a way that somehow functions but is neither elegant nor efficient; the vessels and arteries twisting and curving around each other in a sometimes-baffling randomness. Like those early anatomy lessons in medical school, the interior of Soweto would take me many months to figure out, and many months beyond that before I became comfortable navigating it.

The road I was on suddenly narrowed, and a sun-bleached signpost, tilting at a slightly awkward angle, informed me that Baragwanath was approaching.

Some hospitals tower imposingly over their surroundings; Baragwanath creeps up on you. After driving for a few kilometres along dusty Klipfontein Road, I began to worry that I had somehow by-passed it. Squinting in the glare of the sun, I suddenly caught sight of the small signpost: 'Hospital: Staff Entry'. Braking harder than intended, I veered left, ignoring the stern hoots of the cars behind me. On my right was a gate with a few cars lined up outside. Each car crept slowly towards a small security hut next to a raised boom. No one was stopping, except to ease their cars over the speed bump. Two security guards were chatting animatedly but paying little attention to the traffic crawling past them. They seemed surprised when I stopped and gingerly leaned out my window.

'Excuse me. Do you know where I can park for the medical wards?'

The two guards shared a blank look before staring back at me. I decided to try again.

'I'm ... uh ... Doctor ... uh ... Alastair McAlpine. Today is my first day. I was wondering where the parking lot for the medical wards is?'

A slow grin cracked the face of one of the guards. 'You're new? Welcome to Bara! But please don't steal anything because we check the cars every day before you leave.' He chuckled and I couldn't tell if he was joking or not. 'Don't be frightened. This is a nice hospital and we need the doctors. For the medical wards, go straight, turn right, take the second left, go straight some more, follow the road to right and you'll see the parking lot further along to your left.'

With another hearty giggle, he gently slapped my bonnet, indicating that it was time for me to move on as I was blocking the other cars. I inched my way forward, murmuring the directions to myself, and entered Baragwanath for the first time.

Baragwanath is not like other hospitals. It is not a large and imposing monolith featuring a sleek and sterile exterior. Instead, I was struck by how sprawling it felt. It reminded me more of a run-down suburb in a city than a healthcare facility. There were many single-storey buildings linked by open passageways covered by simple sheets of warped, corrugated iron.

A downcast sign informed me that I was 800 metres from the

PART 1: THE PRESENTATION

medical wards and, as I drove along, I could already sense a thrum of activity; doctors were pacing purposefully to their destinations, car parks were filling up rapidly, patients on stretchers were being navigated through bustling corridors. Although it was only 6:55am, Baragwanath was unmistakably *alive*.

Miraculously, I found the car park, as well as an open parking spot. I pulled in, bowed my head and took some deep breaths. I looked around to make sure no one was looking, quickly glanced down, closed my eyes, and said to a being I wasn't sure existed or not, 'God, grant me the serenity to accept the things I cannot change, the courage to change the things I can, and the wisdom to know the difference.' I got out my car, grabbed my handy shoulder bag, slipped my stethoscope around my neck, and set off for my ward.

As I strode up the concrete passageway looking for my destination, I heard it. It started as a single voice, emanating from the unknown ward I was passing. A lone, evanescent note that lingered before evaporating into the morning air. Before it completely faded, it was augmented by a second, slightly firmer voice, that joined it, lending support to the fragile beauty. Then, like a practised choir, more and more singers joined the melody, harmonising with a practised ease. Startlingly, I could hear singing coming from all directions. I realised that the ward I was standing outside was not unique; *every* ward in this massive hospital was filling the morning air with extraordinary singing.

> Oh Jesus
> You are my saviour
> You are my saviour
> Forever more
> I love you Jesus

My saviour Jesus
I love you Jesus
Forever more.

As quickly as it began, the singing stopped and was replaced by the soft murmuring of the Lord's Prayer. Once completed, a single voice from inside the ward boomed out, 'Thank you, everyone. We are truly blessed to be here. I believe the Lord is watching over us and our patients and will ensure we have a good day. Sister Mathuba sends her apologies: she is not feeling well and will not be coming in. The agency also reported that it was unable to find a replacement for Sister Mlangeni – who is dealing with a family matter – so we will be busy. Important! Please do not forget your tea break! Hypoglycaemia is dangerous and if at any point you feel weak, please sit down and have some biscuits and coffee. First break will be at 10am, with the second at 10:30am …'

My eavesdropping was interrupted by the ring of my cellphone. It was Chloe, my supervising registrar. We hadn't met before and had only exchanged some basic information over the phone. I had agreed to meet her outside Ward 8, the male inpatient ward for my firm, at 7am. I glanced at my watch. It was 7:02.

'Hi Alastair! Just … wondering if you were nearby?'

'Hi Chloe! Yeah, on my way …'

I began marching resolutely, phone clamped precariously between my ear and shoulder. I suddenly realised I had no idea if I was going in the right direction or not.

'Chloe? How do I get to you?' I said. 'I'm outside Ward 14.'

'Keep going up. You'll see a sign at the top showing you where Ward 8 is. If you haven't seen it, continue walking. It's a bit of a trek.'

'Going as fast as I can!' I wheezed.

'Thanks! We have a busy day so best to get going ASAP.'

PART 1: THE PRESENTATION

'Absolutely! I'll be there now-now.' I picked up the pace and tried to keep my beating heart in check.

Medical internship in South Africa began immediately after five or six years of medical school and lasted two years. It consisted of rotating through six different 'blocks', each of which were four months long. Each block featured a different specialty, or a combination of specialties. For my first year at Bara, I knew I would be doing general medicine, then surgery and trauma, and finally obstetrics and gynaecology. The consensus was that general medicine was the busiest and toughest block. Depending on who you asked it was therefore best to get it out of the way early or save it till last. I had decided to dive in the deep end and had volunteered it as my first block.

I had been told I was in the 'Jackson firm', named after the lead physician, Dr Harry Jackson. I once asked why the groupings of wards under a lead physician were referred to as a 'firm', but no one could really give me a reason. 'It's always been that way,' was a common refrain and one I would hear many times over the coming months.

There were five general medical 'firms' at Baragwanath: Jackson, Mpofu, Smith, Mthethwa and Finegold. Each firm was assigned a male and a female ward, with around ninety beds in each. This number was flexible because in times of need, additional stretchers could be wheeled onto the floor. I'd heard that the Mpofu firm had once had over 160 patients in a ward.

Each firm consisted of five interns, five registrars and a medical officer or two. Medicine's hierarchy is strict and confusing to outsiders; its opacity intentional as a way of preserving its order. Like the army, the structure only works if everyone knows their place. Interns are near the very bottom of the physician ladder, with only medical students beneath them. Although we interns were fully qualified doctors, we needed supervision during our apprenticeship. We were not supposed to make any major decisions and had limited prescribing privileges. For this reason, we were paired with a registrar during our internal medicine block.

Medical officers (MOs) were doctors who had completed their internship and worked in a hospital, but had not started specialising yet. The medical officers I had encountered generally fell into one of three categories: the first were those who had just completed their internship and were doing a year of mandatory community service. They were designated as 'COSMOs' (community service medical officers), to separate them from the other MOs. The second group was those gaining experience to enable them to successfully apply for a 'reg (specialisation) post'. Depending on where you wanted to apply, specialty posts were often extremely competitive and time as an MO was essential for your CV. Those in the third group were sometimes jokingly called 'MOFLS' – 'medical officers for life'. These were generally clinicians who were comfortable in their roles and had neither the time nor the desire to put themselves through the rigours of specialty training. In med school, I had learned that the quality of 'MOFL' varied widely; from respected wise owls (who essentially functioned as consultants), all the way to clinicians with extremely questionable knowledge and professionalism. This final group exploited positions that existed as sheltered employment for those who were lazy, incompetent, or both. They rarely left because consequences for their bad decisions were nonexistent, and the perks of extended government service considerable. Soon after I arrived at Bara, a recent audit had revealed that two MOs working in the surgical outpatient clinic didn't hold matric certificates, let alone medical degrees. They had managed to stay employed for

PART 1: THE PRESENTATION

eighteen months because they were hidden in a sea of mediocrity. The hospital barely noticed. From their perspective, a bad (or even fraudulent) MO was better than no MO.

Registrars were doctors who had completed their internship, performed their community service, done additional training as medical officers and were in the process of specialising in a chosen field. Usually, this specialisation took four years. My registrar, according to the orientation package, was Dr Chloe Shephard, currently in her third year. As I strode up the concrete walkway to Ward 8, I wondered about Chloe. First impressions over the phone had been promising as she sounded organised and meticulous. I was petrified about managing so many patients, and I was glad that I would be working with an experienced clinician who could show me how things were done. But a worry gnawed at me. Chloe and I seemed very different and I hoped we wouldn't clash. I knew I could be brash and I had strong views on subjects, which had rubbed people up the wrong way in the past. Chloe was soft-spoken and gave little away. She was precisely the sort of person who sometimes found me overbearing. I also wasn't neat. I had never been neat. I thought my shagginess and disregard for silly details added to my appeal. After all, if Dr House didn't bother with detailed notes when he had diagnoses to make, why should I? I had always considered excessive neatness a waste of time and preferred getting the job done rather than getting bogged down with admin. But exacting colleagues found my cavalier attitude to organisation exasperating, and Chloe sounded *very* exacting. I knew I would have to try to keep things in order, as the key to getting through the early part of this block was to have Chloe on my side. My gut told me that could be a challenge.

I arrived outside Ward 8 slightly breathless, silently cursing the cigarettes and smoking habit I had taken up in rehab. This, combined with sloth-like levels of exercise while I frantically worked my way through mountainous textbooks and files for my final exams, meant that I wasn't in particularly good shape. The long, sinuous corridors already appeared intimidating, but I eventually found the right ward. As I glanced around, I caught sight of a woman in blue pants and a white shirt (the outfit Chloe told me she would be wearing) and waved.

Most kids growing up in South Africa have at one time or another owned a Space Case – a rectangular-shaped plastic container filled with trays and compartments to store pencils, scissors and other stationery. Chloe struck me as the human equivalent of a Space Case: compact, organised, bright, seemingly designed for utility. As she began walking towards me, I noted that even her clipped gait appeared maximised for efficiency. Dark hair pulled back in a ponytail, thick glasses dwarfing her face, her medical bag slung over her shoulder, she seemed neither excited nor disappointed to see me.

'Alastair? I'm Chloe. Nice to meet you. Welcome to Bara. As this is your first day, I decided to come early and see all the male patients first to make it as easy as possible. Here's the list of everyone we're taking care of.' She pulled a few pages from her bag and handed them to me. My heart sank as I eyed the list; it was long and extensive. At least three pages of patient names, handwritten in perfectly ruled blocks, their diagnoses, outstanding investigations and treatment plans neatly listed beside them.

'We got a bit lucky. The New Year period is typically quiet when everyone goes home. We're only on thirty-four. I've earmarked fifteen for discharge today so by the time intake rolls around later, we could be less than twenty.'

'Guess we'd better get to it,' I replied, hoping to sound

authoritative. 'Where can I put my bag? Is there, like, a doctors' room or something?'

For the first time, a glimmer of a smile danced across her face.

'There's a room in Ward 9 where you can leave your stuff. But honestly? It'll probably just get stolen. It's right by the patients' bathroom so they can look in. If they see anything valuable, it's as good as gone. There's a computer in that room for checking results, and some lockers, but they've all been claimed by the nurses and if you want one you need to apply to management. In writing.'

'Is it worth it? Applying for a locker, I mean?'

'You could. I did. Haven't heard anything in three years,' she replied.

'What about just claiming one without a lock on it?'

Chloe shook her head, her face wearing the same expression an adult uses when telling a three-year-old that they can't have all the sweets in the store.

'Alastair. If you claimed a nurse's locker without telling her ... well ...'

She didn't elaborate further; she didn't need to. Chloe had just communicated to me one of the essential, unspoken rules of internship at Bara: never antagonise the nurses. For any reason. They had the power to make your life miserable and it simply wasn't worth it. Ever.

'Let's show you around,' she said.

Baragwanath is one of the biggest hospitals in the world (the third, to be exact), and it felt it. An old army barracks once, it had been awkwardly refashioned to serve as a primary, secondary and tertiary hospital all rolled into one. It resembled a human body in that it was made up of several basic, organ-like brick structures linked by arterial concrete pathways. From a bird's-eye view, I imagined that we all looked like red blood cells, shuttling around chaotically. While following Chloe to the female Jackson ward, I found myself constantly standing aside to make way for stretchers being pushed past. The rusty, oil-deprived wheels made a clanking sound on the rugged, bumpy concrete that the corrugated-iron roofs only amplified. This din drowned out the groans of the prostrate patients as they juddered up and down uncomfortably. Which may have been the point, I thought cynically.

As we entered, I noted that the Jackson female ward was a large open space divided by a single wall and filled with beds lined up next to each other about one metre apart. In theory, these beds could be separated by curtains, but the broken rails and empty hanging clips made it clear that privacy had never been an essential part of the ward design. A few sinks were scattered around the room, many with dripping faucets and brownish basin stains. Yellow sharps containers were pinned haphazardly on the walls, many overflowing with used needles and syringes. The nurses' desk was situated at the front of the ward and a storeroom lay directly behind it (this enabled them to both easily access, and guard, the contents).

As we strolled past the storeroom, Chloe's eyes scanned inside before widening. 'X-ray forms! Grab them!' I wasn't sure what she meant so I stood still, glancing around. With a grunt, she hustled past me and disappeared into the dark room. 'What are you waiting for? Get in here!' I followed her in and saw her reaching onto one of the many shelves filled with everything from scarily large needles to gauze and saline bags. She withdrew a stack of about twenty-five forms and handed them to me.

'These are gold! There's a shortage of forms in the hospital and ordering X-rays without them is almost impossible.' She unzipped my bag and stuffed them inside.

'Why doesn't the hospital make more?' I asked her.

PART 1: THE PRESENTATION

She gave me another pitying look and continued, 'If you ever see anything you need in a ward, grab it immediately. Don't think; just do. If you faff around, it could be gone by lunchtime. It's dog-eat-dog in here and most people have learned to always keep spares in their bags. That includes some basic supplies and forms. You'll have to carry them with you because there's nowhere safe to leave them, and anyway this hospital is too big to be running back and forth. Speaking of which ...' Her eyes quickly scanned the other shelves. She grabbed handfuls of different blood tubes, some suturing material, a few other frightening-looking needles, some blood requisition forms and other paraphernalia I was only dimly acquainted with.

'Here. These should get you through the week. But keep your ear to the ground – there are currently no lumbar puncture needles anywhere. I heard a rumour that Ward 17 had a stash yesterday but my previous intern was eating lunch or something and by the time she got there, they were all gone.' She shook her head. 'Lunch. Rookie error.'

Once I had adjusted to my surroundings, I met the supervising nurse, Sister Ndlovu. She was neatly dressed, her nursing uniform clean and pressed and her maroon lapels firmly affixed. Nurses in South Africa are held in high regard in their communities, and Sister Ndlovu carried herself with obvious pride and with the aura of a respected leader. From my medical student days, I knew that it was essential to get on the right side of the nurses straight away. As they spent the bulk of the time in the wards, I would be relying heavily on them over the next few months.

'Hi, Sister. I'm Dr McAlpine but please feel free to call me Alastair.'

'Thank you, Alastair. I'm *Sister* Ndlovu.' There followed a slightly awkward pause but she didn't say anything more.

Chloe chimed in, 'Sister has been at Baragwanath – and in the

Jackson firm – for nearly twenty years. Isn't that right, Sister?'

'Nineteen and a half,' she confirmed with evident pride.

'Wow! You must have seen a lot of interns like me in your time,' I said.

'Oh yes. You youngsters arrive with your shiny clothes and think you know everything. More than the nurses. A few months here sorts you out.'

'Well ... I'm here to learn!'

'Deal with the patients first. Then you can learn.'

'Okay ...'

'Work hard and be polite,' she continued. 'We learn very quickly who the rude, young doctors are. We know how to deal with them ...'

Chloe took this moment to grab my arm. 'Thanks, Sister! We'll let you know if we need anything!' With that she scooted me away down the hallway.

Now that I was 'orientated', it was time to see patients. Chloe and I went together to see the first one: an elderly woman who had suffered a stroke. Her name was Mrs Dlamini and Chloe started going over her history and treatment. I nodded, acting as if this were completely normal and not the first patient I had ever seen in my life as an actual doctor. While she was going through the plan, my mind zoomed back to all I had learned about strokes in medical school. The hours I had spent memorising the long list of causes; how to elicit the precise location of the stroke in the brain through a thorough neurological exam; how the management of these cases was complex, requiring not just medications but rehab, physiotherapy, speech therapy, education on prevention of further strokes, and close follow-up. My mind was a blur and by the time Chloe got to the end, I realised I had hardly taken anything in.

'So. We've started her on aspirin and a statin. I've also added another antihypertensive agent as her blood pressure was 196/104 on arrival. This is the fourth drug she'll be on for her high BP, but she's not all that compliant, so ... we'll see. Don't get your hopes up. She seems to have settled, but her family say they can't take care of her, so we're waiting for placement at a step-down facility.'

For the first time since arriving in the ward, I glanced at our patient from the end of the bed. A short, frail woman was sprawled out in front of us. She was clearly not aware of our presence and her gaze roamed haphazardly around the ward, as if searching for an anchor to tether to. One side of her face and body drooped; both were unresponsive. An IV line was attached to her right arm, connected tenuously to a 1-litre bottle of saline fluid. The site around her arm was worryingly swollen and I mentioned my concern to Chloe.

'Ah, shit,' she exclaimed. 'It's tissued and no longer in the vein. She needs a new line or else she'll dehydrate – this one isn't drinking anything. Think you can just re-site it?'

In an attempt to impress Chloe, I responded, 'Uh, sure. No problem,' and immediately regretted it. I had inserted a couple of IV lines as a medical student, but these were always under supervision, on patients who were in reasonably good shape with big veins and who had consented to being jabbed by a nervous trainee. Here, there was time pressure *and* I was being watched by my registrar.

I knew this was a test of sorts; Chloe was deciding how competent I was and how much she could trust me going forward. The temperature in the already hot ward felt like it had gone up five degrees.

Chloe opened her bag and laid out a new IV cannula, an alcohol swab and a transparent plaster. First, I needed to remove the old cannula. I tried, as gently as I could, to detach the dirty sticker covering the entrance site. Other than a slight grunt from Mrs Dlamini as it came off, this went smoothly. I exhaled and tried to wipe away some of the sweat that had accumulated on my eyebrows and was threatening to drip down onto the patient. As I had gloves on, I had to use my elbow to try to wipe it away, and only managed to smear it more efficiently over my forehead. I bent down again to remove the cannula, which was surrounded by hardened, swollen flesh, courtesy of the fluid that was no longer flowing through a vein and had leaked into the surrounding tissue. I put a piece of gauze next to me on the bed, ready for when the old cannula came out, and gingerly pulled.

The minute the plastic cannula came out, two things happened simultaneously: her arm started bleeding profusely from the exit wound, and the cannula, now free from the pressure it had been under, began spurting saline.

'You didn't close the drip?' Chloe's voice sounded both startled and annoyed.

'Shit! No, sorry! Shit!' With one hand I jammed the gauze over her arm, hoping to stop the bleeding. With the other, I tried to grab the IV line that was leaking fluid onto the floor around the bed. Chloe reached it first and stopped the flow, but I found myself standing in a puddle of saline.

'Sorry,' I stupidly muttered again. Then looked down at our patient. 'I'm sorry, Mrs Dlamini.' She was frowning as if aware that she was in fumbling, inexperienced hands.

'Okay, Alastair, we're running behind. Can you get the new one in?' The bleeding, mercifully, had stopped and I quickly applied a dressing.

I grabbed a tourniquet out of my bag and walked around to the other side of the bed. I slid it around the patient's arm and tightened it. Her thin and frail arm did not have a lot of subcutaneous fat on it, so to my relief a bunch of veins popped up nicely. I identified the biggest and straightest one I could find, which happened to be in

PART 1: THE PRESENTATION

the crook of her elbow (the 'cubital fossa' as I had learned) and set about cleaning the area with an alcohol swab. Once it had dried, I unsheathed the IV cannula from its cover.

The cannulas used in hospitals are different sizes, ranging from extremely tiny for newborn babies, to much larger ones for adults. The one I was holding was green and a typical size for an adult. At that moment, it looked like a hosepipe to me. I wondered whether I should swallow my pride and ask Chloe for a slightly smaller pink one, but she was busy with her notebook and I felt like I had something to prove. Gritting my teeth, I palpated the vein, which seemed to slide from my fingers at the slightest pressure. Every time I brought the cannula close to the vein, it shimmied away, as if frightened. Eventually, I took the plunge and slipped the cannula through the surprisingly tough skin. The patient groaned briefly but otherwise remained still. To my relief, I saw an immediate flash of blood in the cannula's window, indicating I had hit a vessel. At this stage, the aim was to slide the plastic cannula over the needle into the vein. Practised physicians do it in one smooth motion with their index finger. I was not confident enough yet, so I used my right hand to anchor the needle in place and my left to slide the cannula in. It wouldn't budge. I tried again, but still nothing. I tried to withdraw the needle, leaving the cannula in place, but as soon as I did, the area around the cannula immediately swelled with blood. With a heavy heart, I knew what I had done. I had gone straight through the vein. Now it was ruined.

Blown IV lines happen all the time, but I wanted the ward to swallow me whole. I was the new intern, on his first day, standing in a puddle of saline, gloves covered in blood, with disappointed looks from both the registrar and the patient boring into my skull.

Once Chloe had expertly sited a new line in about thirty seconds flat, and restarted the IV fluids, we moved on to the remaining patients. I tried to remember all their names, and some of their details, but soon they all began to blur. By mid-morning, I could no longer remember if Ms Tshabalala in bed 8 had meningitis or acute kidney injury; if Ms Mahlangu had gout or pneumonia; if Mrs Ndlovu had hypertension or diabetes. The 'to-do' list piled up rapidly: a dozen chest X-rays, five ultrasounds, two new CT scans of the head and at least ten patients who needed their bloods sent to the lab. My bag continuously slipped off my shoulder as I tried to balance the forms I was filling out, my list of patients, the small pocket textbook I was frantically trying to read between cases to bolster my knowledge, and the notebook of outstanding tests required. I was becoming flustered and frustrated. Chloe sensed my distress and stopped.

'Don't stress too much about feeling overwhelmed on your first day. But to get through this place, you're going to need a system. Do the stuff early that can't be done later. Take X-rays, for example. They're done on a "first come, first served" basis so get the completed form to the department when you arrive in the morning. Arriving a few minutes earlier than today wouldn't hurt ...

'Bloods are done by a ward phlebotomist so those requests should be in the tray by 9:30am. Having someone else take your bloods is a godsend! But if you miss that deadline – like today – you're on your own.

'Consults to other services should be done before lunch time. Wait till after that and people get grumpy and might not come, which means you'll have to call them again the next day. Remember: *everyone* is totally overwhelmed and looking for any excuse to defer your question or consult. When you do get hold of someone, try to speak to the registrar NOT the consultant. The registrar is newer and less confident and is less likely to refuse to come.

'CT scans and MRIs require a direct chat with the radiologist. We have two CT scanners; one runs twenty-four hours a day, the other runs twelve. They are always fully booked, even for emergencies. To get your requests approved in this place you sometimes need to … "massage" the truth a little bit.' She saw the slightly confused look on my face, so she grabbed my list. Her eyes darted down until they settled on a name.

'Here, for example. Mr Mbuza needs a head scan to make sure he doesn't have an abscess in there. If you just write "Bacterial meningitis. Slow recovery. Needs scan to exclude an intracranial collection", the radiologists will respond "Only if he has abnormal neurological findings" and turn you down. Now, Mr Mbuza's level of consciousness has *technically* remained unchanged …' She paused, a small glint in her eye that I had never seen before, 'But I didn't see him move his eyes earlier. Did you?'

'No, I guess I didn't …'

'Exactly! So you write on the form: "Eye movements not detected". That should do it.'

'But wasn't he just sleeping?'

'Who cares?! The radiologists don't know that. They get bombarded with requests daily so they're really strict about who they'll scan. If there isn't a good reason, they'll image someone else instead. And our patient really does need it. Understand?'

'Okay …'

'Sometimes they may want to speak to you, to try to see what's what. Stick with what you wrote down and don't give an inch. He needs a scan.' She saw the nervous frown flit across my face. 'Don't worry. You can tell them whatever. It's not like they're going to come and examine the patient themselves.' She thought this was funny and laughed and then glanced down at her watch. 'Shit! We're behind. Let's go.'

After finishing up the remaining patients, Chloe informed me that our firm was on intake for the day. This meant that for twenty-four hours, any patient who needed admission to the general medicine wards came to the ones in the Jackson firm. The intake started at 7am and ended at 7am the next day. All patients were seen first in the emergency department (ED), and if deemed sick enough, sent to the relevant service for admission. All adults with general medical illnesses came to Ward 30, where we took a history, did a thorough exam, performed what tests we could, and then decided, based on how sick they were, whether they needed to go to the ICU, the high-care area, or the ward.

Ward 30 is notorious. A lone building with an unassuming exterior, its fearsome reputation has spread to all four corners of South Africa. Like any medical student, I had heard the stories, which were as frightening as they were harrowing – long lines of patients, limited resources and a race against a ruthless clock. Nevertheless, walking in, I was initially underwhelmed. It felt like a large warehouse with very thin cardboard walls that didn't quite reach the roof, separating it into different cubicles numbered #1 to #5. Each cubicle had four to six beds and its own stock of supplies. I saw a reception area with five collection trays, one for each cubicle. Our tray already had eight patient folders thrown haphazardly on top of each other. These were patients who had arrived while we were busy in the ward. Part of the reason Chloe was in such a hurry was to avoid arriving too late and being unable to clear the backlog.

Two bored receptionists sat in front of a large admission book, fanning themselves. The tattered pages were full of small squares under the number of each cubicle. Every patient who came in was assigned sequentially to a cubicle until the row was full and then the process would begin again. There was a queasy randomness to this system because you never knew what the next folder contained or

PART 1: THE PRESENTATION

how sick the patient was.

The firm was divided into 'teams' that consisted of either a registrar and an intern working together, or a medical officer working alone. The number of teams that worked by day and by night was left entirely up to the firm, however there was an element of strategy involved. With a total of six teams, the division of labour was important. Put five teams on during the day to handle the bulk of the patients but risk managing the evening with a single night team? Or provide extra coverage at night but expose the day teams to a higher workload? The stakes were high. A few nights before, the Mpofu firm had risked a single night team and the poor registrar and intern duo had been completely overrun, admitting over sixty patients. We heard that the post-intake ward round only ended at 6pm. To avoid a repeat of that our firm had decided to approach that day's intake with four day teams and two night teams. Chloe and I were one of the day teams so this meant we would be seeing every fourth patient. We were randomly assigned cubicle #3 and while we were settling in, she gave me a brief tour of the ward.

'Welcome to Ward 30. It's busy here. Duh. You already knew that. I'll be able to help you in the beginning, but ultimately you'll need to pull your weight 'cos it's too much for me on my own. Cubicle #3 is okay – it's got a bit more space than the others but the bad news is that we're next to psych.'

'Psychiatry? They're here as well?' I asked.

'Ja. See that cubicle over there?' She pointed to the only one that had a gate separating it from the rest of the ward. 'That's psych, who also use this as an admission ward. Sometimes we get called there if they want a medical referral. If they even sniff a non-psychiatric cause for a patient's psychosis, you'll be there doing all the work for them. Be warned: you can't take any sharps in there – someone got stabbed with a needle just last week.' I was shocked and waited for her to elaborate, but she continued as if she had simply given me a weather update. 'Also, no drips. Patients sometimes try to strangle each other with the fluid lines.' The same matter-of-fact tone, which was somehow more frightening than if she had emphasised the horror.

'The gate is to stop patients escaping?'

'Sort of. If they really want out, the exit is nearby. Dudes escape all the time. The main reason is to stop them causing havoc in the medical cubicles.'

'They do that?'

'Oh, sure. Last month one of them got access to the specimen box.' She pointed to a large wooden tray in the centre of the ward filled with clear plastic bags containing blood and fluid specimens from patients. This box was the common drop-off point for all the cubicles.

'For some reason this patient decided to drink all the tubes containing cerebrospinal fluid. God, what a pain. We only found out the next day when the lab told us all our specimens were insufficient.' She shook her head and walked on.

'This final cubicle is high care where the acutely unwell patients go. Don't worry, it's managed by the registrars, so you won't have to do anything here. I'll probably be back and forth between it and our cubicle. You're not required to go there but if general medicine is your thing it's where the seriously cool pathology goes, and I'd be happy for you to have a look.'

I went back to our cubicle and placed my bag in the corner where I could keep an eye on it. My stomach, which I had not noticed until now, began grumbling. Chloe hadn't even mentioned lunch and was hastily going through the folders, so I figured it wasn't the time to bring it up.

I decided to look at some of the referrals and took a few of the files designated for our cubicle. Initially, I thought there had been some kind of mistake. On reviewing the notes from the emergency department all I saw was: '35 y.o. male, p/w (presents with), cough. DDx (differential diagnosis), pneumonia or TB'. That was it. After squinting to see if there was anything I had missed, I took the file to Chloe.

'Oh ja. That's Dr Mbindwane, alright. She's notorious for this stuff. She works at Chiawelo Clinic by day and moonlights here at night and on her days off. Lord knows when she sleeps.'

'Does nobody care about the quality of the referrals?' I asked.

'Not really. Proper clerking and examination are considered our job. And Mbindwane can see, like, thirty patients in an hour. She pushes that queue like nobody's business, which gives the other doctors a chance to breathe and do their jobs. Without her, that place would be overrun.' She grabbed the remaining files and quickly scanned them.

'Here,' she said, handing one to me. 'This looks like a reasonable start. Overdose. Get going and let me know when you're done. I'll start on another.' I paused for a moment as something struck me – this would be the first patient I had ever clerked in as a doctor. I had trained and studied and dreamt of this moment for years and now, with no fanfare, it had arrived. That odd sensation of experiencing something that was both incredibly important and somewhat banal overcame me. I glanced down at the name: 'S. Mtombini. 46 years old. Overdosed on unknown tablets. No other medical Hx (history). For investigation'. I flipped through the rest of the notes to get more information, but those few words seemed to be it. Some vital signs had been done in the ED showing his blood pressure was a bit low at 98/75, but nothing to panic about. I approached his bed gingerly.

'Uh. Good evening, sir. My name is ... uh ... Alastair. I mean, Dr McAlpine. But you can call me Alastair if you wish, I'm not fussy.'

The patient didn't move so I continued, 'I'm an intern here and I'll be looking after you. Can you tell me what brought you in?'

Mr Mtombini was curled on his side in the fetal position, facing away from me. His body was rigid and when I touched his shoulder, he retreated into himself, like a tortoise entering its shell seeking protection from an outside threat.

'Mr Mtombini? Sir? Can you tell me what's the matter?'

At this moment, a harried-looking nurse shuffled in. Glancing at the patient, she clicked her tongue in a way that conveyed both disapproval and concern at the same time.

'Mxm. That one. He's been here before. Always trouble with the wife. He drinks too much and then takes too many Grand-Pas. Then he calls the ambulance.' She approached him, leaned in his ear, and muttered, 'Mtombini. Hayi wena! You can't keep doing this. This hospital can't handle marital problems in addition to all the HIV.' Then hearing a soft sob that emanated from the form on the stretcher, she straightened up, clicked her tongue again, shook her head, and left to assess the next patient.

My mind was a whir of thoughts. Grand-Pas. Headache powders that contained aspirin and caffeine. If he had overdosed on aspirin the acid-base levels in his body could be abnormal. I cast my mind back to the toxicology lecture in med school. Part of my brain concluded he would have too much acid in his body and another part insisted he might have too much base. While the warring factions in my head battled it out, I decided to take some blood to make sure. Chloe seemed absorbed with her own work so I grabbed a syringe and a needle. Just in the nick of time, I remembered that a sample for the blood-gas analyser needed to have heparin, an anticoagulant, in it to stop it from clotting and damaging the machine. I grabbed the heparin bottle, pulled some into my syringe, moved the plunger back and forth, and then hesitated. Do I leave the heparin in? Or do I squirt it back out? If I squirt it out won't the blood just clot? I decided to trust my gut and left a bit in at the top of the syringe. Ready to make my first real diagnosis, I approached Mr Mtombini.

I thought I needed a sample from an artery for the measurement to be accurate and so I told Mr Mtombini what I was planning to do, and that it would hurt. He whimpered and cowered further into himself, but he did not resist when I extended his arm and began feeling for the radial pulse just above his wrist.

Possibly due to his anxiety, his pulse was rapid but the cool sweat that coated his body meant my fingers kept slipping and losing their grip. I bit my lower lip and committed to inserting the needle.

Mr Mtombini yelped and tried to pull his arm away. I managed to maintain my grasp and felt massively relieved to see bright red blood filling the syringe. I filled a few extra tubes too, before removing the needle and pressing a piece of gauze down hard on the bleeding.

My one hand was now holding the exposed needle and tubes, and in the other I was attempting to staunch the bleeding. I glanced around, cursing myself for not checking where the nearest sharps disposal was before starting the procedure. My eye caught on the bright yellow container ... but it was two beds away. I tried to ease the pressure on his wrist to see if I could make a dash for it, but blood immediately began oozing from beneath the gauze. In a panic, I considered throwing the needle at the sharps container but quickly realised this was both dangerous and stupid.

'Drop the needle, Doctor.' It was the nurse from earlier.

'Sorry?'

'Drop it. Then cover it with your shoe.' Seeing the scepticism on my face, she continued. 'It's safe. That needle can't penetrate the rubber of your sneakers and it's lying on its side so you're safe from the sharp bit. That will free up a hand to tape the gauze down.'

'We were always told this was dangerous.'

'Have you got a better idea right now?'

I slowly dropped the needle, made sure it wasn't sticking up, and then slid my foot over it. Once the gauze was taped down, I bent down and picked up the needle and disposed of it in the sharps bay. I knew I had broken about a dozen safety rules regarding sharps but I didn't care. At least I hadn't stuck the needle into the side of the bed, like some of the interns I had watched as a student. I hurried over to the blood-gas analyser and inserted my sample.

After two minutes of whirring and humming, the machine spat out a small piece of paper. I had a look and gasped. It was as I thought – his body had become too acidic in response to all the aspirin. In addition, his sodium levels were worryingly high. Brandishing the proof in my hand like a winning bingo card, I approached Chloe.

'Chloe ... my patient who overdosed? He's pretty sick. Check this out.' I handed her the printout. Her eyes widened.

'Shit. This is surprising. I thought he looked pretty good, but obviously I was wrong. He's going to need high care. Did you take this gas yourself?' I nodded nonchalantly, as if this were routine for me.

'Okay, good, I'll get a bed ready. Tell the nurses to bring him through.' With that, she hurried off to prepare.

After Mr Mtombini was settled in high care, I exhaled. That was a good catch. My instinct had been right. Perhaps I was cut out for this after all. I permitted myself a brief smile, before grabbing the next folder from the pile that seemed to be growing rapidly.

While busy with my next patient, Chloe came through to the cubicle, her forehead perplexedly crinkled. 'Alastair, could you run me through how you obtained that arterial blood sample?' I could feel my pulse quickening. I went over what I had done, but the more I talked, the deeper her frown etched into her face. My brain began short-circuiting. Had I clotted up the machine? Had I interpreted the results incorrectly? Had I not acted fast enough and now my first patient was on a downward spiral to inevitable death, followed by a hospital inquest into the intern who took too long to diagnose him?

None of the above, it turned out. Chloe sighed wearily. 'Alastair. You're not supposed to leave the heparin in the syringe. It messes everything up. I know because I repeated his blood gas and it was completely normal, except for the hyperventilation you caused by stabbing his wrist.' I felt my neck become warm. The cubicle suddenly felt unbearably small.

'You didn't trust me?'

Chloe sighed. 'I trust you but you're an intern. It's, like, your default to mess up. That's why I'm here, to find your errors. "Trust but Verify," that's my motto. You should make it yours, too.' She then scuttled off to continue the work. I needed a cigarette. Badly. But the patients were piling up and I didn't want Chloe to think less of me than she already did.

It was when our eighth patient was wheeled in with a red 'urgent' sticker on his forehead that I knew things at Bara were different.

'Why does he have a sticker there?' I asked the nurse.

'Because he's sick, Dokotela, and needs to be seen urgently. If the sticker went in his file, no one would notice.' In its crazy way, the logic made sense. I opened his file and saw a urine dipstick stuck onto the first page, proving he had ketones in his urine.

Right at that moment, Chloe walked past and started ranting. 'I've never understood why they feel the need to include the actual dipstick, with patient urine on it, in the folder. They should just write what it showed – I'll believe them! I'm just glad they don't include the glove when they report blood on the rectal exam ...'

I started clerking the patient and trying to manage his diabetic coma from all the acid in his body. I was unsure whether I should remove the sticker from his forehead or leave it on. I decided to leave it, and no one, including the patient, appeared to notice or care.

I don't remember much about the other patients I saw that first day, except their names. I remembered those. I recall that there were so many of them and there was so much work to do. Very little had been done in the emergency area and if we were lucky they came with a chest X-ray or an IV line.

It quickly became apparent that med school had not prepared me for this, and the template we had used for seeing patients (thorough history, followed by detailed clinical exam, followed by appropriate investigations, then a differential diagnosis and treatment plan) did not apply at Baragwanath, especially in Ward 30. There was not enough time. Patients were wheeled into our cubicle whether there was space or not. We had to treat the urgent stuff, do the relevant tests, and get them to the ward. Fast. Chloe jumped around, nimbly examining and scribbling notes, while I fumbled and tripped over gurneys, IV stands, personal belongings and shuffling nurses. As soon as one patient was dealt with, another one filled their place. Each one was sick. Each one was in pain or distress. Trying to treat them as individuals when they all merged into one amorphous blur became increasingly difficult.

I managed as best I could, trying not to make any major errors. I finally managed to get some IV lines in, which boosted my confidence. I was exhausted, but time was passing and it felt like we were making some progress.

Our cover was due to end at 11pm, sixteen hours after I had arrived, when the evening teams would take over. At 10:30pm, following a merciful lull, the doors to the ward flew open and the whole world arrived at the same time.

By this stage, Chloe and I had admitted twenty-seven patients. My feet hurt, my back hurt, my eyes were red from the fluorescent lights, my lips were cracked and chapped from the dry highveld air, and all I wanted was to sit down. For just thirty seconds. I would have sold a kidney just for the briefest of respites. The last time I had yearned for anything like this was when I had gone fishing with my father and brother and became horrifically seasick on the huge swells. I remember thinking that I would have done anything – anything at all – for the boat to stop its sickening lurching. Just for a few seconds. Now I had a similar sensation, but this was driven by fatigue, not nausea. Ward 30, however, was not known for easing interns in gently.

'All for us?' I squeaked at the porter. At this stage, it felt like the day was descending into a farce. Surely this couldn't be right? *More patients?*

'Haha, yes, Doctor. We have to take our dinner so they build up a bit while we eat. But here they are!' With that, he and his team distributed the stretchers between the various cubicles and left.

I realised I had not even had time to meet the other interns and registrars I was going to be working with in the Jackson firm. The day had passed by so quickly that there simply hadn't been a minute to spare.

When confronted by this overwhelming mass of people, all of whom needed my help, it suddenly hit home how horribly ill-equipped I was. Trying to manage this tsunami of suffering felt as futile as trying to staunch the incoming tide of the ocean. I couldn't do it.

Waves of self-pity rolled over me, bringing hot tears to my face. I rushed to the corner of the cubicle, hoping Chloe wouldn't notice, but while I was staring at the wall, taking deep breaths and trying to compose myself, I heard a voice behind me. It wasn't gentle but it wasn't condemnatory either.

'Alastair, it's tough here. This is how it goes. Feeling overwhelmed is part of it. Get some fresh air, grab something to drink. I'll make a start. Come back when you're ready. But the most important thing is to come back.'

I considered not coming back. I considered getting in my car and driving home and never returning. As I gulped huge breaths of air outside, I felt a tap on the shoulder.

'Try this. You'll feel better. Some sugar and caffeine will help.' A kind male voice behind me draped a can of Coke over my shoulder. I started with a few sips, which grew until I was greedily sucking down huge gulps, overcome by a thirst I hadn't felt for years, a thirst beyond one of simply hydrating the body. For a moment, I was reminded of the thrill of downing a beer; the warmth that emanates from the stomach, the blissful drift towards oblivion.

I turned around to thank the kind soul who had given me the drink but they were gone. The sugary Coke and fresh air calmed me down. I glanced at my watch. I had nearly survived. Only fifteen minutes to go.

I turned around and re-entered Ward 30.

Time seemed to draw out more and more slowly as we approached the blessed end of the shift. Chloe emphasised that it was important we didn't leave unfinished work for the night teams unless absolutely necessary. As the clock struck 11pm, a cry came from reception, 'Slate closed!'

I slumped into a chair, too shell-shocked to really know what had just happened. I had sweated through my shirt and even my shoes felt damp. The hunger I had suppressed all day (both lunch

PART 1: THE PRESENTATION

and dinner had passed by with barely a thought) suddenly began gnawing at my intestines, and I felt like I had walked into a wall of sudden nausea. I put my head between my legs and tried to take some more deep breaths.

Chloe's neat Converse sneakers clipped into view.

'It's done. Now, I know it doesn't feel like it, but we got a bit a lucky today. It's still holiday season for most so numbers weren't as bad as usual. We'll be presenting all our new patients to Prof Waters tomorrow. He's a stickler for results so make sure you have them all handy. Here, take these.' She handed me a sheath of paper.

'Rounds start at 7:30am. It'll probably take you about an hour and a half to get all the results from the computer, so you'll need to be back here by 6am. Computers are available on a first come, first served basis and can be found in the lounge back there.' She gestured vaguely behind her.

'See you tomorrow!' Her demeanour was friendly enough, but we both knew today had been a test. And it felt like I had failed.

Chapter 2
A NURSERY OF INTERNS

JUST AS CHLOE HAD SAID, ROUNDS WITH PROF WATERS STARTED PROMPTLY AT 7:30am the next day. I had been so tired the night before I could barely remember driving home, but when I had finally crashed on my bed after filling my stomach with a bowl of pasta thoughtfully left in the microwave by my mum, I hadn't been able to sleep.

My heart was beating uncontrollably and every time I closed my eyes, I visualised the patients I had seen that day. Mr Mtombini and the unnecessary tests I had exposed him to because I had been too stupid to empty the syringe and too proud to ask for help; Mrs Abrahams, whose blood tubes my quivering hands had dropped and whose medical details I could no longer remember. There were so many.

Suddenly, bile rose in my throat and I bolted to bathroom where I vomited up my dinner. Washing my mouth out, I looked in the mirror. The image staring back seemed to have aged five years in one day. I wasn't sure I could do this, but eventually fatigue overcame anxiety and I drifted off into a deep sleep.

I dreamt of a frail arm covered in oozing sores. As I curiously touched one, it bloated beyond all recognition, bursting saline fluid as it ruptured. Instead of screams there was giggling around me; helpless, uncontrollable giggling that erupted into mirthless guffaws. I looked around to see who could be making a mockery of such an awful situation, but no one was there. While I searched angrily for the disrespectful joker, I abandoned the frail arm, which promptly dropped lifelessly to the floor. When I turned back, all was black, and I was lost. The laughter turned into shrieks, until I had to cover my ears. I awoke in a cold sweat as the sun was beginning to rise.

Prof Waters was a distinguished-looking man in his sixties. His white, shining hair was neatly clipped and combed back over a head showing the faintest signs of baldness. His medical coat gleamed like a newly whitened tooth, and he walked with the coiled, elastic energy of a man dedicated to lifelong exercise.

After polite introductions ('You studied in Cape Town, eh? Always preferred Wits graduates myself.'), we started reviewing the patients in the ward.

Finding the patients earlier that morning had turned out to be a lot more complicated than I expected. While each firm was assigned a male and a female ward, due to the sheer number of admissions, these wards often filled up by 6 or 7pm on intake days. The 'overflow' patients were then redirected to any other ward where there was bed space. None of this was computerised so I had to go to every medical ward in the hospital and manually cross-check my admission list with the nurses' book of patients currently admitted. Worryingly, I had not been able to find Mr Mtombini. I wanted to see how he was recovering from his overdose.

I went to talk to Chloe about it in Ward 30, but she was looking harried and stressed, darting between her patients in the high care, adjusting knobs on machines and fiddling with infusion rates, all of which looked impossibly complicated. I couldn't bear the thought of appearing even more foolish in her eyes so I resolved that come what may, I would find Mr Mtombini on my own.

Unfortunately, by the time rounds started I still had not been able to locate him, and further questions to the nurses and ward clerks elicited blank stares. Eventually, Sister Ndlovu asked if I had checked the 'small book'. Seeing my confusion, she pulled me closer to her, glanced around, and then whispered, 'It's where we put patients who, you know ... go to the second floor.'

'I don't understand,' I responded stupidly. 'There isn't a second fl–' I caught myself just in time but Sister Ndlovu's eyes had already rolled back so far in her head I could only see the whites.

The possibility that Mr Mtombini might have died had never occurred to me, but now I broke into a cold sweat. Please let me not be the intern whose first patient died on their first day, I silently prayed. What would my colleagues and Prof Waters think?

Sister Ndlovu unlocked the small drawer in her desk and took out a tatty, disconcertingly well-thumbed book. I swept through the pages, searching for this week's deaths. Scaling up and down the names with my eyes, I nearly fainted with relief when I couldn't find Mr Mtombini's. He was alive, I just had to find him.

'Ms Jacobs is a sixty-four-year-old woman who presented with a cough and shortness of breath for three days. She is a non-smoker but has a history of TB fifteen years ago. Co-morbidities include hypertension and Type 2 diabetes, for which she is on hydrochlorothiazide and metformin. She takes no other medication.

'Vitals were as follows ...'

'Ahem.' A small cough from Prof Waters interrupted my presentation. Disconcerted, I looked at Chloe who was standing impassively.

'Uh. Vitals were ...'

'Ahem.' Louder this time. I looked up from my notes. The professor was looking at me like a slightly disappointed parent. 'What's a "vital"?'

'I don't understand, Prof.'

He sighed. 'Young man. Precision in medicine is important. That extends to our language. There is no such thing as a "vital". "Vital" is an adjective. I presume you meant to say "vital *signs*"?'

'Uh, yes. Of course. Sorry. The patient's vital signs were as follows: saturations of 89% in room air but 98% on two litres of nasal-prong oxygen. Respiratory rate of twenty-four breaths per minute, which makes her tachypnoeic. There was a fever of 38.8 degrees Celsius. Blood pressure was 148/93. Blood glucose was 12.9.

'Examination revealed a somewhat emaciated elderly woman with generalised, shotty lymphadenopathy, especially in the neck and axillae. She was neither clubbed nor was she cyanosed. Auscultation of the chest revealed ...'

'Ahem.' I looked up again. 'Firstly, lymph nodes are not *shotty*. "Shotty" is not a word you will find in any dictionary, medical or otherwise. Secondly, patients are not *clubbed*. If they were they would be in the trauma ward with a head injury. They *have clubbing*. How exactly did you assess for this?'

I briefly explained how I had examined the end of the patient's fingers, looking for a pulpy expansion and an abnormal angle between the nail bed and the cuticle. This sign is rare, but often heralds more serious lung and heart disease.

Prof Waters was listening to Ms Jacobs' chest with his stethoscope while placing her opposite fingers together, nail to nail, and positioning them in front of the light from the nearby window. His brow furrowed; he told me to have a look. No light could be seen between the fingers.

'Now try it with yours,' he instructed. Sure enough, when I did, a tiny diamond-shaped gap was visible between my fingers.

'That's Schamroth's sign!' he exclaimed. 'Named after Prof Leo Schamroth who was a physician at this very august institution! He described it in himself when he unfortunately came down with endocarditis. You won't read about it in fancy textbooks but this patient has it!'

The triumphant tone was unmistakable and for the first time that morning, Prof Waters smiled.

'This patient likely has a lung abscess. Get a CT scan and when it's confirmed, call the surgeons. Keep her on broad-spectrum antibiotics in the meanwhile.'

'But ... how do you know? I haven't even told you my examination and X-ray findings yet.'

'Let me guess. Bronchial breathing in the right middle zone posteriorly and X-ray shows a consolidation in that area?'

'Uh ... yeah. That's amazing.'

'Also, exclude TB. And do an HIV test! I do it on everyone. Let's move on.'

'But, er ... what about her social history? I really think it has a bearing ...'

'We can't save the world, Alastair. We are clinicians. Our job is to fix the problem that brought her in. We have social workers and such for the other stuff. We simply cannot solve every social ill in greater Soweto.'

I glanced helplessly at Chloe, who seemed to have found something interesting on the floor to draw her attention. I looked back at my scribbled notes with the sharp, untidy handwriting that slanted drunkenly across the page. I had noted that Ms Jacobs had recently lost her partner to a rapidly progressive stomach cancer. He

PART 1: THE PRESENTATION

had been a kind man and the Jacobs' family only source of income. Ms Jacobs had dedicated her adulthood to raising their three children. His death, and the subsequent depression that followed, had acted like a tiny puncture on the tyre of Ms Jacobs' health, with her spirit sighing away almost imperceptibly in the weeks and months after his funeral. Her diabetes, which was previously meticulously managed, was now out of control, and had almost certainly contributed to the development of her lung abscess. Her next appointment with her GP was over two months away and it felt like we needed to address this issue more urgently. But Prof Waters and Chloe were already on their way to the next patient. I made a mental note to follow up on Ms Jacobs' case and chased after them.

As we were walking to the next patient, Prof Waters strolled next to me and began musing. 'What would you call a collection of interns? A kindergarten? A nursery? Medical collective nouns are a bit of a hobby of mine, you see. Some seem quite obvious. A "shitload" of proctologists, for example. Or a "school" of paediatricians. I'm an endocrinologist so it's a bit trickier. A "gland" perhaps?'

'A "secretion"?' I suggested drily.

'Oh! I like that! A "secretion". Yes!' And he drew out a small notebook from one of his many pockets and began writing it down. Fortunately, the collective noun for interns he was looking for appeared to have disappeared from his memory.

After a few patients, I began picking up a few things about Prof Waters. He was a brilliant, but impatient clinician. This may have been because routine illness and disease posed no challenge to his intellect and therefore bored him. Or it may have been because he ran a private clinic at a different hospital in the afternoon and was impatient to get there. Or it may have been that after many, many years at Baragwanath, he was simply burnt out and tired.

He was a repository of fascinating information about the hospital. At one point, between patients, he asked if I had seen the marijuana field. When I could only respond with a confused stare, he laughed.

'There's an entire marijuana field behind the staff parking lot. An oasis amongst the drudgery, you could say. It's strangely beautiful and the plants somehow manage to stay cultivated. No one knows how or by whom.' The briefest of smiles indicated that there was only one possible candidate. 'It's one of this hospital's best-kept secrets. Let's try to keep it that way, eh?' And with the briefest of winks, he marched ahead.

As the ward round proceeded, we spent less and less time with each patient, until, at around midday, Prof Waters glanced impatiently at his watch, and asked, 'How many more?'

'Three left.'

He glanced at Chloe. 'Any of them complicated? Any uncertainty about the management?'

'No, Prof,' Chloe responded with confidence. I was somewhat surprised, given that at least one of the remaining patients was *very* complicated, but I stayed silent.

'Good, good. Thanks everyone. Strong work,' and with that Prof Waters powered off.

'Okay, Alastair,' said Chloe. 'I think there's plenty there to keep you occupied. I have teaching this afternoon, but if you need any help just let me know. I need to see my supervisor about my research project. Take fifteen and go say hi to the other interns over there.' She nodded at a group of friendly-looking doctors huddled together under one of the few real trees in the concrete jungle of Bara.

Grateful for some company, I sidled over.

PART 1: THE PRESENTATION

'Hey! There he is! The final member of the team!' A large hand, attached to a stocky guy with thinning hair and a generous smile, extended out to greet me. I shook it generously. I recognised the voice from the previous night, the one that had kindly handed me the Coke.

'Alastair.'

'Kobus, and these here are Angela, Anwar and Phelo. I think we're it for the Jackson firm.'

Angela was tall and striking, her red hair in stark contrast to her pale skin. She smiled demurely and held out her hand.

Anwar had curly hair and was sucking generously on a cigarette, which made me suddenly crave one.

'Got a spare?' I enquired.

'Help yourself. Kobus? I know the look of a hungry smoker when I see it. Want one?'

Kobus paused. Then he glanced around, 'Why not? My wife hates it when I do ... but I guess she's not here, is she?' he said with a chuckle.

With the ice broken, we began chatting. Anwar was from Durban and had studied there. He was at Baragwanath because he had been 'second-rounded' and hadn't matched with any of the hospitals closer to home. He said he was a 'city boy' and that Jozi felt like the next logical place if he couldn't get Durbs.

Kobus was from Pretoria ('Tuks of niks!'). He was newly married, with his first child on the way. He had the assured air of someone acquainted with their own strengths and limitations.

'I leave all the specialisation stuff to the smart people,' he stated confidently. 'I just want to get through this and be a GP.' His wife had a job near the hospital so he had moved to be close to her. Kobus was an open book; he said what he meant and always got straight to the point. But it was clear that there wasn't a malicious bone in his body and he enjoyed the role of court jester. I liked him immediately.

'Anwar, got another smoke?' Kobus asked as soon as the first one had been greedily sucked down.

Angela had remained engaged, but quiet throughout, smiling at Kobus's good-natured jokes. I asked her about herself and why she was here.

'Oh, I don't know. I'm a Witsie. I studied here. I know the place. I suppose I just thought, "Why not?"'

There was a brief silence as we digested this unusual reason for coming to Bara. There were plenty of other options for Wits students who wanted to stay in Johannesburg, and this hospital was too intense for all but the committed. 'Why not' seemed strange, but then again so did Angela.

I decided to change the subject. 'How are your consultants? I got Waters. He's smart but a weird dude.'

'Yeah, he was like that in med school. Keep patient numbers down and he'll be happy,' Angela added. 'I've got Simpson. Pulmonologist who smokes like a chimney. Ironic. Fun but overly familiar with his female trainees.'

'Ugh, isn't he married?' said Anwar.

'Ja, but it's on the rocks. He was having an affair with one of the registrars and his wife found out. Wasn't the first time either.'

'It all sounds a bit gross,' I chimed in.

'It is ... but he's also one of the few consultants who doesn't always look like he'd rather be elsewhere. He really does care about the patients, so ... pros and cons.'

'I've got Khan,' Phelo said. 'He seems okay.'

'One of the smartest consultants at the hospital,' Angela replied. It was becoming clear that she had her finger on the pulse of the Bara staff. 'But in his off time, he runs an alternative medicine practice.'

'What, like, homeopathy?'

PART 1: THE PRESENTATION

'Homeopathy, Ayurveda, naturopathy ... you name it, he's probably got some kind of master's degree in it.'

'You better watch out, Phelo. Sounds like you're going to be prescribing herbs and crystals in your post-intake rounds!' Kobus said.

'Nah, you'll be okay,' Angela calmly responded. 'He doesn't mix his disciplines. World-respected rheumatologist by day, alternative healer by night. Don't know how he squares that in his brain, but he manages.'

'I know exactly how he does,' said Anwar, flinging imaginary dollar bills our way.

'Hey, have any of you guys heard about the marijuana field?' I asked.

Angela smiled again.

'Oh ja. It was planted a few years back by Prof Waters. Or so we think. If you keep an eye out long enough you'll see him visiting. How he manages to keep it hidden, I'll never know. If the patients found out it would disappear overnight.'

'Do you know where it is?'

'Sure. Follow me.' Angela walked off and those of us who were smoking threw our butts on the floor and jogged after her.

After a few minutes of navigating the fences at the back of the parking lot, and ducking under some trees and through dense shrubbery, we saw it.

I don't know what I was expecting, but this wasn't it. In amongst the weeds and unkempt vegetation, an area the size of a squash court had been lovingly cleared. Within it a neat crop of marijuana plants stood withering under the harsh sun. It was clear that they had been planted and maintained with intent and skill but the heat at this time of year was simply too intense.

'It's ... beautiful,' Anwar said, with the admiration of a man who knew his weed.

'Can we take some?' Phelo asked out loud.

'This wouldn't get you very far,' Anwar responded. 'It's dry and shrivelled but maybe after some rain ...?'

Before the idea could percolate among the group properly, my phone rang. It was Sister Ndlovu. A patient's family was in the ward and wanted to see me.

'But it's not visiting hours,' I responded, checking my watch. Those were between 3 and 5pm.

'These aren't usual visitors,' she said.

'What do you mean?'

Her voice dropped to an ominous whisper, 'Just come, please.'

'Okay, I'll be there soon, I'm just finishing up something.'

'Please Doctor, they're gangsters. Come *now*.'

On my way to the ward, my heart thudded and multiple thoughts jostled in my brain. The first was that this was *not* what I had signed up for. Soweto could be a dangerous place, especially in the wrong parts, but I had always thought we were safe within the hospital walls. The fear in Sister Ndlovu's voice told me that this was not the case. I tried to phone Chloe for back-up but was transferred to her joyless voicemail. I groaned. In our psychiatry block we had learned how to deal with violent patients, but there had never been a lecture on how to approach violent *family members*. As I raced to the ward, I realised that I didn't have a plan.

By the time I arrived, a sizeable crowd had formed around the bed of the patient concerned. I remembered him vaguely from the previous evening. An elderly gentleman who had come in confused, likely due to pneumonia. We had started him on antibiotics and oxygen, and he seemed a bit better on rounds, although still disorientated. It was likely that he would need at least a few days of

PART 1: THE PRESENTATION

treatment in the ward before we would consider discharging him.

I made my way through the crush of nurses and patients that had formed around his bed. Two huge men dressed in matching jeans each had two imposing guns tucked into their belts, and were pulling leads and cords and the oxygen mask off the patient. He was sitting up, looking a bit dazed, but repeating over and over, 'I want to go home ...'

I approached the men with what I hoped was an air of calm and authority, but I was very frightened. I hoped my voice didn't betray my fear.

'Good morning. I'm Dr McAlpine. I'm the intern looking after this patient. Can I help you?' is what I hoped I would say.

'Uh ... er ... Hi! What's going on here?' is what I actually said. Or squeaked.

'Are you the doctor?' An imposing and intimidating voice from one of the large men silenced the entire ward immediately. It was a voice that commanded deference through the implicit threat of violence.

'I ... am. What can I do for you?'

'This is our father. We're taking him home.'

'But ... he's sick. He has an infection in his lungs and he's old. Without proper treatment, it could get worse.'

'Voetsek, wena. We're leaving.'

At that moment, my phone rang. It was Chloe. I nearly fainted with relief. I walked to the side and answered.

'Alastair? What's going on?'

'Chloe? Where are you?'

'Just with my supervisor ... Dr Simpson. Sorry, it went on a bit long. What's up?'

I tried to explain the situation as best I could as I watched the elderly gentleman yank out his IV line, which then caused his arm to bleed.

'Doctor! Come sort this out,' the one intimidating man ordered. Before I could react, a nurse hurried in obediently and placed a gauze over the exit site. 'I don't want you. I want him,' he growled, nodding at me.

I raised my hand to try to buy myself some time while I explained the situation to Chloe.

'Whatever happens, you can't let him leave. He's confused. He cannot sign a red slip.' I glanced over and saw that he was, in fact, writing on a red slip the nurse was holding in front of him. 'Just keep them occupied. I'm on my wa–' Before I knew it, Chloe's voice was gone, along with my phone. One of the men had grabbed it and was tucking it into his pocket.

'You don't talk when my father is bleeding. You fix it.' The humiliation burned, but I didn't see what choice I had. One of the nurses thrust some gauze and a plaster into my hand. I approached the elderly man who was trembling and looking around like a bewildered cat.

'I want to go home ...' he mumbled.

'Okay, okay. I understand. Let me sort out that arm, okay? We don't want you bleeding out before you make it to the parking lot.'

Once the gauze was secure, I turned again to face the men and cleared my throat. 'I need my phone back now. It's essential for other patients.'

The man who had taken it drew it out like a blade and slapped it into my hand.

'Thank you. Now I know you say he wants to go home but I don't know that your dad is in a state to sign that refusal of medical treatment form.' I was pointing at the red slip.

'Fine. He won't sign it. But we're still leaving.'

'I don't think that's a good idea ...'

PART 1: THE PRESENTATION

The man glared at me. 'What are you going to do about it?'

At that point, a nurse shuffled up to me. 'Just let him go, Doctor. Please! We don't want violence. Some of us live in the same community. He and his kids are bad men. Drugs, alcohol, cigarettes. We don't want to upset them.' She then lowered her voice to an almost imperceptible whisper. 'Maybe it's not a terrible thing if he gets worse ...'

I looked into her eyes and saw no guilt, only fear.

At this point, the three men were getting ready to leave. They walked over to me imposingly, their brute physicality in stark contrast to my medical authority. It was clear who wielded the power, despite this being a hospital. I could try to impede their progress, perhaps call security, perhaps make a fuss. It was clear that leaving was not in the patient's best interest, but this had escalated to a point way beyond my level of authority.

I stepped aside and let the men pass. As they exited, the ward seemed to exhale, and I crumpled onto a chair. A few minutes later, Chloe arrived, red-faced and sweating. She had clearly run to the ward. I'm not sure who was more upset, me at her for taking so long to arrive or her at me for letting a sick patient leave. We stared at each other for a while, then, shaking her head, she wordlessly left the ward.

By 4:30pm I was in real trouble. My 'to-do' list was glaringly incomplete, but with many services winding down for the day some items would have to wait until tomorrow.

Everything was taking longer than anticipated. Blood draws were painfully slow, IV lines needed replacing at an alarming rate, and patients and their families seemed to have endless questions that I didn't know the answers to.

By 5:30pm, Anwar waved me over to share a cigarette.

'How's it going, man?' he asked jovially.

'Jesus. I'm buried. How about you?'

'Totally fucked. But I'm broken and going home. We try again tomorrow.' He flicked the cigarette away. 'It's a marathon not a race, dude. There will always be more work.' With that, he slung his backpack over his shoulder and started walking towards his car.

'Hang on. I'll follow you.'

It felt like I had hardly made a dent in my list of patients, but I was feeling the fatigue from my brutal first day and the very early start that morning. Every task I completed seemed to throw up two new ones (a call to a surgeon required another X-ray and additional labs; a switch in antibiotics required an ECG and consent form). I was never going to finish everything so I grabbed my bag, walked to my car and dumped it in my boot. I hoped Chloe wouldn't see me leaving.

Approaching the exit behind Anwar, I saw a cloud of dust and then a long queue of cars waiting to exit. I briefly wondered what the hold-up was, but my brain was too tired to really care, so I stared out the window and tried to let my thoughts settle. This was the first time in nearly 48 hours that my mind wasn't whirring at a 100 miles an hour, and I enjoyed the sensation of just *being*.

As I approached the boom gate, I saw the security guards stop every car ahead of me and search them thoroughly ... including the boot. When it was finally Anwar's turn, I saw him open his and so I popped mine without a second thought. I couldn't wait to get home.

After a minute or so it became apparent that something was wrong. It was taking too long, and I could see movement at the back of Anwar's car. There was a lot of rummaging around and some vague gesticulating. Eventually, the concerned face of the security guard beckoned Anwar to get out of his car. He stepped out and was confronted by the guard holding his bag, open, with its contents exposed. Like me, Anwar had accumulated various items from the hospital over the past two days. These included forms, blood tubes, needles, catheters, blades, glass slides and other equipment. The security guards' preoccupation with Anwar meant they hadn't got to me yet and, with a jolt, I realised what was going on.

I leapt out of my car, sprinted around to the boot, grabbed my bag, and hurled it into a nearby bush. Hoping neither of the guards had seen me, I jogged over to join Anwar.

'Doctor. What's this?' It was the same guard who had warmly greeted me the day before, but the joviality of the previous morning was gone. This voice was stern. Anwar was being interrogated.

'Uh … just stuff I need to do my job, you know? The wards aren't particularly well stocked sometimes so we just kind of …' I could see the guard's face darken, '… grab stuff.' I could tell that Anwar blurting this out was a mistake.

'But it's not yours. You can't take it home. This is theft.'

What had struck me a few minutes ago now dawned on him. 'What? Oh! Oh god no! It's not *theft*. I'll be bringing it all back tomorrow.' The guard raised his eyebrow quizzically.

'You could be selling it, Doctor. There's a black market.'

'What? No! Why? Who would I even sell this stuff *to*? It's not like I have a side hustle or anything!' He chuckled desperately, trying to lighten the rapidly darkening mood around him, but his attempt at levity failed.

'Doctor, we warned you and all the young doctors about theft yesterday.' He turned to look at me for the first time. 'Didn't we, Doctor?'

Anwar's face collapsed. He looked like someone standing on a trapdoor that had unexpectedly opened beneath him.

I tried desperately to negotiate. 'Look, surely we can work this out? There must be something we can do? Maybe a warning? He won't do this again, will you, Anwar?'

He shook his head vigorously.

'I'm sorry, but we have no choice. You'll need to come with us,' the guard said.

'Come with you? Where?' Anwar's voice had dimmed to a hoarse whisper.

'To the police station.'

'You can't be serious.'

'Don't make us arrest you. We can sort it all out there.'

A bizarre thought suddenly crossed my mind (and Anwar told me later he thought the same thing): could he be spending the night in a Sowetan prison? For an innocent stash of hospital equipment? It all felt so surreal.

We decided not to cause a scene. He called his parents while I contacted Chloe, who assured me she would speak to the relevant people and sort it out as soon as she could. Then I jumped back in my car and followed the security van with Anwar in it to the nearest police station.

In the end, he was let off with a warning. The police had bigger fish to fry than a bemused junior doctor with some hospital equipment of minor value in his bag. He was told sternly not to do it again and as I walked back to my car, I saw the grinning face of the security guard.

'Sorry, Dokotela, but we have to get the message out there somehow.'

I realised that the guards knew this would happen. They knew Anwar would face no serious consequences, but they were using him as an example to other interns. It was all just a stunt. I wasn't sure whether I was more angry or shocked. After giving Anwar a hug, I got back in my car, slammed the door and drove off.

PART 1: THE PRESENTATION

I drove past a petrol station and found myself making a rapid U-turn and pulling into the parking. Although I had never been to this particular garage before, I was in a routine that felt as natural as breathing. The trembling anticipation. The thought of the taste on my tongue. The crack of the can as it opened with a soft hiss. I grabbed two large energy drinks, paid, and almost sprinted back to my car. The first went down with sickly ease; the rush of sugar and caffeine following shortly afterwards. The trembling ceased. The voices tearing through my head calmed. I opened the other can, took another large gulp, and finally headed home.

Chapter 3
CERTIFIED

I CONTINUED TO CHECK ON MS JACOBS AND A FEW DAYS LATER SHE WAS A LOT better. The CT scan had confirmed the abscess in her lung and it was responding well to antibiotics. She was sitting up in bed, joking, and chuckling amiably. Her fever and chest pain had both settled and the nasty cough was dying down. Encouragingly, her breakfast tray was empty. I didn't need six years of medical school to know that a return of appetite was a promising sign.

'Doctors, thank you! I feel much better.'

'My pleasure,' I responded. This felt like my first real win, and I was going to enjoy the moment.

'So ... you know ... now that I'm feeling better ... when can I go home?' She giggled as she said it, using the levity as a shield in case our response was negative. Chloe glanced at me so I responded, 'Well. You see. This is a serious infection. Although you're feeling better, you'll need a long course of antibiotics. We're also going have to try get that diabetes under control or this could happen again.'

'But, Doctor, I must get back to my kids. I can't stay here forever. Can't you just give me the tablets?'

PART 1: THE PRESENTATION

'I'm afraid it's not that simple. We're not ready to discharge you just yet ...' I was interrupted by her sobbing.

'I hate it here,' she said. 'It's dirty and smelly and old. I don't sleep at night and it's noisy during the day. I miss my family. Please can I go home?'

At this point, Chloe stepped in. 'I'm sorry, but no. You need to trust us on this. If you go home early, you may get sick again and die. And your family wouldn't like that, would they?' There was an awkward pause before the sobbing resumed.

'Let's move on, Alastair. She'll come round. It's for the best.'

My list wasn't getting shorter and I was spending too long with each of my patients. By the time I got to radiology to book my scans for the day, it was nearly 4pm. I would have asked Chloe to help, but she was with her research supervisor again. Going there alone I knew my chances were slim, but I had to try anyway. As I rounded the corner, I heard a voice steeped in honey.

'So, look, I know it's a bit cheeky, but if you could just squeeze her in, I would be soooooo grateful!' Then I saw her. A band of colour on a sheet of grey. The first thing that caught my eye was the platinum-blonde hair, cascading down her back, ending almost at her hips. Most colleagues with long hair kept it in utilitarian ponytails, as free-flowing locks tended to get in the way of procedures and exams. There were also plenty of surfaces you didn't necessarily want your hair to brush against, so this was unusual. It was also dyed so light that it almost illuminated the notoriously dark radiology rooms. A striped-red shirt hugged her slim figure and emphasised her long legs, over which she had squeezed a pair of jeans.

'Okay, Mandy, I'll see what I can do.'

'Tom, sweets, you're the best!'

'But you're pushing it! Next time you're going to have to let me take you out.'

'Oh, Tom! I'll pencil you in!' And with that, she winked and whirled around, her hair following in a perfect parabola, and nearly crashed straight into me.

'Whoops! Sorry! Didn't see you there.' A beautifully made-up face with sharp features glanced at me. This lasted for a split second before it broke into a wide grin revealing slightly disjointed, imperfect teeth.

'Haven't seen you round before,' she said playfully, before placing her hand nonchalantly on my arm. Ostensibly to move me aside, her touch felt probing instead. 'Handsome interns are a rarity in this place.' With that, she winked again, and strode off.

I shook my head, as if waking from an afternoon nap, and approached the radiologist.

'Hi! I know it's a bit late, but I was wondering if I could book some scans?'

'Sorry. Bookings closed for the day.'

'But you just made one for … Mandy, I believe? Is there something I'm missing?'

He glanced at me as if I were a blind rat and then went back to his documents. I sighed audibly, but the radiologist remained unmoved. Walking away, I vowed to return first thing the next day. I could still feel the burning sensation where Mandy's hand had touched my arm.

That evening was my first overnight 'ward call'. On top of my regular day, I had to stay overnight to monitor the wards and complete the tasks organised by the day teams, but that could only be done at night. As there was just a single intern covering eight hundred inpatients, ward call was a daunting prospect.

The shift technically began at 5pm but by 4:30 the calls started

PART 1: THE PRESENTATION

rolling in. Mr Mpangeni in Ward 6 needs his blood transfusion at 10pm, Ms Skosana in Ward 9 needs her insulin levels checked at 8pm, Mr Zondi in Ward 17 needs to have his renal function tests drawn at 7pm ... The list went on and on and while it was exhausting zooming around the hospital, there was a sense of satisfaction to be gleaned from the small tasks successfully completed. I had a list, and with every unit of blood I hung up, every dose of medication adjusted, a duty was crossed off and the list became shorter.

By 11pm it was looking likely that I would be able to sneak to the intern room to get some dinner and possibly even lie down for a few minutes. At that moment, my phone went off. It was a nurse from one of the other medical units in the hospital – the Smith firm.

'Doctor. There's a patient here. She's bleeding. She's not well. Can you come?'

'Where is she bleeding from? How much blood?'

'Just come, Doctor.'

Medical school had taught me that when experienced nurses call, you listen. I grabbed my bag and my stethoscope and hurried to the ward. The nurses saw me and gestured to a bed with the curtains ominously drawn around it. The atmosphere was eerily silent.

I grabbed the patient's file and quickly perused it. Her name was Lily and she was twenty-three, two years younger than I was. She had a bleeding disorder, the details of which were unknown despite extensive investigation. She had not responded to any of the treatments given to her and was unable to form any clots. This meant that she was at high risk for bleeding spontaneously, which is exactly what was happening. Her blood pressure was low and her IV line was no longer working. I also noted that due to her poor prognosis (euphemistically reported as 'guarded' in the notes), she would not be considered for ICU admission.

This felt like something way above my pay grade. I gulped and opened the curtains. I saw a person lying there who, in a different set of circumstances, could have been a friend of a friend I met at a social braai. Despite being clearly unwell, her skin still had a youthful sheen, and she mustered a gentle smile as I entered.

'Thank you for coming.' Her voice was so faint it felt like it was ebbing away between each word, like water running through fingers. There was blood oozing from her nose and down each arm from previous puncture sites. I quickly checked her pulse, which was rapid and weak. An automatic blood pressure machine was positioned next to her bed. It showed that her blood pressure was worryingly low, probably from some internal bleeding.

The truth then hit me: Lily was dying.

I quickly phoned the on-call ICU registrar, who took her details before asking the patient's name. When he heard my response, he sighed. 'Ja, we know her. She's not for ICU. Her prognosis is so poor and we have no beds. She's not for CPR or anything like that. Just try to make her comfortable. Get up an IV line, give her some fluids and maybe some morphine.'

I went back to Lily who opened her eyes with difficulty. The nurses had, while I was on the phone, brought the equipment I needed for an IV. I snapped on my gloves but my heart sank when I applied the tourniquet. Her body was shutting down from the blood loss and trying to conserve flow to the central parts of her body. As a result, the veins in her arms were all but impossible to detect. The only visible ones were smallish vessels on the top of her hand. I moved the tourniquet down her arm and flicked her wrist, more in hope than expectation that a suitable vein would reveal itself. When none did, I closed my eyes and offered a silent prayer.

As I was grasping her wrist, looking frantically for a vein, I felt a warm, gentle pressure in my hand. Her fingers had closed around mine. It was a simple gesture and I immediately looked into her eyes. I will never know if it was the case, but I think she saw the desperation of a junior doctor trying to do something – anything – in the face of the inevitable and wanted to comfort me. She offered a consoling smile, grimaced, and then whispered, 'Doctor, I'm afraid. Can you stay here and hold my hand?'

By this stage, blood was seeping from her nose and lips, and her breathing had become laboured. I needed to act; I couldn't just stand there.

I let go.

Rushing back with another IV cannula, I tried for a vein on the other hand. I got it first time. As the line slipped neatly into place and I connected the cannula to a bag of fluid, she sighed, looked upwards, and died.

In death, finally, Baragwanath offered privacy. Curtains were drawn; space was provided; deference was shown. An invisible, but palpable barrier surrounded the beds of the departed, and there was a solemnity that enveloped the space like a blanket.

One of the jobs of the overnight call is to certify the dead. Only a doctor could do this and it had to be done before the body could be taken to the morgue. When Lily died, I robotically went through the motions. I gently checked if she had a pulse in her neck. Nothing. I listened to her heart. Her chest was still. I checked her pupils, which had begun to glaze over. They were fixed and unresponsive to light and when I touched her eye, she had no corneal reflex. The look on her face was neither peaceful nor pained. She simply appeared as if she had been in the process of taking a deep breath and had then … stopped.

I closed her eyelids with my hand and offered a silent apology for not being able to do more. Then I started scribbling in her file but stopped. What was an appropriate note to write? 'The patient demised'? That seemed very cold. Ditto for 'The patient expired'. Despite spending only fifteen minutes with her (was it really only fifteen minutes? It felt like an eternity and a millisecond rolled into one), I felt a connection to Lily. I knew, in her final documentation, that she deserved something more personal, so I thought about it and then wrote, 'At 8:57pm, Ms Lily Makhubula passed away. May she rest in peace.' I had no idea whether that was better or worse, but I didn't have time to dwell on it; my tiny moment of peace was interrupted by the ringing of my phone. It was another ward, with another patient needing my attention. I got up to answer it, and then made my way to the next task. I began to realise that grief was not an emotion Baragwanath gave you time to dwell in.

I certified five patients that night, which was considered normal for a ward call. I had been told that there was no need to rush these certifications, especially after 11pm, as the morgue was closed and only opened its doors at 5am. Whether you certified someone at 11:01pm or 4:59am, they would remain in the ward. Most of us quickly learned to begin 'certification rounds' at 4:30am, but potentially earlier if there had been more deaths than usual.

After you've certified dozens of patients, you realise a few things. The first is that to be around someone who has died is to occupy a sacred space. Breath has become air, blood has separated into water, joints have frozen, eyes have glazed. You are with a vessel that has completed its journey, and all that remains is its legacy. Whether that legacy is, like a fallen trunk in a forest, something that nourishes others, or, like ash in a fireplace, something that disappears with the wind, only the living can know.

The second is that there is a *warmth* to the living, generated by more than just body temperature. It is as if the spirit, or the soul, acts as an internal furnace, generating the heat that powers life. When this furnace is extinguished, the human body becomes not just cold, but *frigid*. Life has not just ended, it has completely vacated the space. To touch a dead body is to be acutely aware that death is not just the absence of life, it is the complete antithesis of it. It is a humbling reminder of how fragile we all are and how precious the tiny flame of consciousness we all possess really is.

I once asked Chloe why we didn't attempt to resuscitate more patients. She responded that the wards were so poorly stocked, and many of the patients so chronically ill, that 'resuses' rarely succeeded. Should you manage to stabilise someone, there was still the very real possibility of there being no space in the ICU. Anwar had discovered this the hard way on his first call. He had managed to intubate a patient and was pumping oxygen into her lungs when he was informed there were no ventilators in the ICU. To his credit, Anwar manually bagged air into her lungs for six hours until one was found. For his trouble, he got berated for intervening without checking with ICU first.

Angela had told me that on her first night on ward call she had been called at 3am to certify someone in one of the distant orthopaedic wards. She was wide awake and had no other tasks so she went straight to the patient. The nurses expressed surprise at her rapid arrival, but wearily pointed her to the appropriate space. When she opened the curtains, she saw immediately that the elderly gentleman was alive, but gasping for breath. Confused, she went back to the nurses' station to check she had the right bed. When it was confirmed, she told the nurses that she could not certify the patient because he was still alive, albeit in a critical state.

'Hawu, Dokotela ... this is what happens when you come early ...'

I left work the next day at 6pm, thirty-five hours after arriving. I remember climbing into my car and everything spinning around me. An overwhelming sense of fatigue, which I had been keeping at bay, suddenly settled on me like a cobweb. I promised myself I would only close my eyes for a moment ... but when I opened them, it was dark outside and three hours had passed. I knew I needed to get home but every movement felt leaden. I drove to the local petrol station and bought two Red Bulls and a coffee. I splashed some water on my face from the bathroom tap and then tried to take a large gulp of coffee but ended up pouring it all down my front. The adrenaline jolt was a weird relief because I knew the hazards of driving home in my state.

I downed one of the Red Bulls, savouring the jolt in my bloodstream, then opened the other. I wound all my windows down and cranked the A/C as strong as it would go. I slapped my cheeks a few times until I felt ready and then gingerly began the drive home.

Every doctor who has driven home after a particularly long overnight shift knows how treacherous that journey can be. The hypnotic blur of the lines on the road, the soft whirr of the wheels, the gentle rumbling of the engine, all combine to convince you to close your eyes. Just briefly, no big deal. Unless you are actively turning the steering wheel, shifting gears, or doing something to stay alert, the eyelids inevitably droop. This makes any stop, or any stretch of straight road, particularly hazardous. I knew how unsafe it was to drive, but I didn't have a choice – there was no other way to get home, and all I wanted was the sweet oblivion of sleep. I gritted my teeth, felt the cold air on my face, and focused all my might on keeping my eyes open, blinking only when my eyeballs ached.

Miraculously, I arrived home unscathed. I could barely force a few spoonfuls of soup down my throat before passing out into the deep, dark comfort of slumber.

'Hi, handsome.' A hand, soft as a whisper, brushed my shoulder. 'Wasn't expecting to see you here.'

The slight twang of Afrikaans, blended with the huskiness of vocal cords dusted with cigarette smoke. Even in the dark environment, inflamed by the methodic beats of the DJ and the gyrating bodies of healthy, attractive twenty-somethings, she stood out. Her platinum hair perfectly groomed, a slight sheen of sweat indicating she had recently been on the dance floor.

'Oh, hi Mandy! Didn't know this place was your scene.'

She raised an eyebrow quizzically and leaned in. 'After the week I've had, I needed to blow off a bit of steam. Some wine. Some dancing. I think we all need it. Also, thanks for helping me out with that turf. I believe I owe you one.'

My initial joy at seeing her was replaced with slight irritation that the first thing she had brought up was work. At Baragwanath, if a team discharged a patient and that patient was readmitted within one month, the admitting physician could 'turf' them back to their original team. The earliest I had come across the phrase was in Samuel Shem's controversial *The House of God*, where interns were encouraged to 'buff and turf' patients to other specialties. Ostensibly to ensure continuity of care, 'turfing' a patient became the easiest way to reduce your patient load and receiving an unexpected 'turf' was one of the least pleasant ways to start your day. Mandy had somehow managed to convince me to receive a turf even though it had been my predecessor who had discharged the patient. I still wasn't sure what had possessed me to accept.

It was three weeks since we had met and this was my first precious weekend off. In the landscape of internship, a weekend when you're off from Friday night to Monday morning is called a 'golden weekend'. Although this was a misnomer because the truth is they were worth far more than gold. After nineteen straight days at work it felt priceless. Our group of interns had decided to go to one of the more popular nightclubs in Johannesburg, Manhattan. My offer to be the designated driver had been gratefully accepted by Anwar, Phelo, Angela and Kobus.

We had arrived at the club an hour or two earlier. I had heard Mandy would be coming, but seeing her beautifully dressed up in a short skirt caused my neurones to short-circuit. Meanwhile, she had stretched over the bar, pushing herself onto the tips of her toes to provide just slightly more elevation than everyone around her. It worked. A bartender rushed over, even though there were clearly other people who had been waiting longer.

She glanced at me and winked. 'Two shots of vodka, please.'

'Mandy, uh, no. I can't drink it.'

'Oh, stop being so straight for once. This isn't Baragwanath.' By now she had paid and was holding a shot glass towards me. For just a moment, I considered it. No one would know. I was tired and desperately did not want to have 'the chat' with Mandy, whose interest in me seemed to be ebbing away with every passing second.

'Yeah, I know,' I responded. 'But I can't.'

'Why not?'

Briefly, I considered telling her the truth, but tonight I wanted her sexual interest, not forensic curiosity. In that moment I did not want to feel as if I were a specimen on the dissection table.

''Cos I'm driving.' I was relieved to have a plausible – and true – excuse.

'You're not leaving anytime soon. One won't put you over the limit.'

'I'd just rather not, y'know?'

'Oh well, more for me then.' She knocked back both shots in quick succession, gave me a weak smile, as if I were a pet to be pitied, and sauntered off in the direction of the dance floor. I couldn't take my eyes off her as she disappeared in the roiling mass, until a hard thump on my back broke the spell.

'That chick is trouble, bro.' Anwar's slightly slurred voice was both beer-infused and solicitous. 'She's only interested because you're a challenge and she doesn't understand you. But she'll use you and spit you out. Girls like that always do.'

'You're being harsh, man. She's never done anything to me.'

Anwar raised an eyebrow sceptically. 'It's already happened, dude. I overheard that turf she sent your way. That patient had been discharged for nearly two months! By someone else! No way was it your problem!'

'She said she didn't know.'

'What? *Everyone* knows the rules for turfing. It's like ... Bara Etiquette 101.'

'I guess ...'

'She does this with everyone. That cute smile. The long hair she flicks at all the right moments. She's a tease and she uses it to her advantage. That one radiologist? He refused a scan for my dude who fell off his bed and cracked his face on the concrete floor. "Let's be real, Anwar, he's no oil painting. A scan won't change that." That's verbatim, by the way. But her patient who got hit by a bloody *tennis ball*? CT scan that evening. He wasn't even on call that night but he did it as a "favour". She's bad news. Watch out.'

I glanced back at the dance floor and Mandy was shaking and writhing, encircled by a group of men eyeing her like a pack of hyenas. In irritation, I looked away. Within a few minutes, Angela, Phelo and Kobus had rejoined the group.

'Mandy over there has her hooks in Al,' Anwar announced, pointing with his beer. Kobus seemed a touch jealous while Angela eyed me with the pitying look of someone who had seen this sad movie play out before.

'Oh, Al,' she muttered. 'Men are so predictable.'

Changing the subject, I announced that the next round was on me. This was met with cheerful enthusiasm. Everyone, it seemed, was looking to blow off some steam.

I ordered the drinks and when the bill arrived, I couldn't help but notice that a few beers and glasses of wine cost more than many of my patients earned in a month. The contrast between the abject poverty I saw by day, and the extreme, casual wealth I was surrounded by at that moment was so glaring it was impossible to ignore. I had been to Manhattan before, but never after spending nineteen straight days with people who were so poor that some couldn't afford shoes on their feet. It felt gaudy and garish, but I tried not to dwell on it. I just wanted a break – to relax and dance and not think about Baragwanath-bloody-Hospital, and my list of fifty patients, for just a few hours. After all the suffering and death, I wanted to bask in the aura of health and vivacity, the shiny flesh, the beautiful bodies, the lack of disease.

I wanted to get lost and forget. We all did. I couldn't rely on the alcohol, but there were other ways. I downed an energy drink and immediately felt the familiar jolt to my body. I glanced around and saw an intern in another firm had joined our group. I had seen her around but had never introduced myself.

'Who's that?' I whispered to Phelo, trying not to be too obvious.

'Who? Her? Oh, that's Lucy. She's in the Finegold firm. Why?' He paused, then smiled. 'I see what you're up to. She's single. Go dance with her, man!'

I – again – decided to change the subject. 'Phelo, after the week we've had, how come you look so chilled? How do you do it?'

He languidly finished his beer and glanced at the bottle. 'Work smart. Not hard.'

'It's impossible not to work hard where we are.'

'Ja, well, you can make your life easier, or you can make it harder. Which reminds me ...' He tried unsuccessfully to grab the attention of a nearby waitress. He turned back to me. 'Anyway, you gotta find a way to make your workload manageable. Otherwise, you're never going home. Arrive on time in the morning, work hard, and unless someone is dying, bail at 5pm. No one is paying us for overtime and there is *always* more work.

'Fix the problem the patient came in with and get them out. We can't be solving everyone's complete medical needs. If some other problem is severe enough, they'll come back and you can sort it out then. One problem per new patient and move on.

'Speaking of new patients, when you get one, go through their chart with a fine-tooth comb. Find out who the previous doctor was. Turf them back to that doctor whenever you can. Continuity of care and all ...' He burped. 'But if someone tries to turf a patient to *you*, do whatever you can to avoid it. Claim you were on leave and didn't sanction the discharge; or claim the month was written wrong. Whatever. But just avoid turfs. We have enough work without doing other peoples'.

'Speaking of which ... know who's got the whole "get others to do work for you" vibe?' He pivoted around and his gaze fell on Mandy. 'That girl over there has it *sussed*! Just the other day she tried to get *me* to do a lumbar puncture on one of *her* patients. Said she had tried and failed multiple times but when I had a look, she had just stuck a plaster on the patient's lower back! No puncture marks! And the worst part is, knowing I was being duped, I *still* fucking did it! Some people, man ...'

He noticed that I was eyeing out Lucy on the dance floor. He sighed, grabbed my shoulder, and looked deep into my eyes with the maudlin intensity of the very drunk. 'Lucy's cool, Al. If you're just gonna use her to distract yourself from Mandy, find someone else. She deserves better.' He let off another belch. 'Now, I'm going home. My taxi's ready. Ward call tomorrow. Gotta catch some Zs.' With that, he tipped his bottle down his throat, making sure every drop was drained, and then walked slightly unsteadily out the club.

By this time Lucy was looking over and gave me a flicker of a smile. She chose that moment to raise her arms and sashay her hips to the deep hip-hop blaring from the speakers. Her shoulder-length, brunette hair splashed over her face and the strings of her dress stretched taut across her clavicles, like wires waiting to be cut. At that moment, her enthusiasm was something I wanted to get lost in. Phelo had a girlfriend; he could sermonise to someone else. I smiled back and walked towards her.

When, after three songs, we found ourselves next to each other, my arm on her waist, she leaned in. 'Fancy seeing you here.'

'Fancy seeing you here yourself.' It wasn't my smoothest line but she smiled anyway.

'Shouldn't you be dancing with Mandy?' she said.

'Why would I be doing that?'

'Just seemed like you were into her.' I glanced over to where Mandy had been, but she was now in the arms of a tattooed hulk who was running his large hands all over her body, to her obvious delight.

'Fuck Mandy.'

She smiled. 'Right answer.'

Hours later, with dawn breaking, we stumbled out of Manhattan. The group of Baragwanath medics had been the last people to leave the club to chants of 'One more song!' every time the DJ threatened to stop playing the music. It was as if, more than anyone else, we were unwilling for the respite to end; we needed the night of freedom and excess to carry on before another week of work started again. Lucy

PART 1: THE PRESENTATION

and I had been kissing non-stop but despite endless energy drinks, we were both beginning to feel the inevitable crash coming. I half-heartedly asked her if she wanted me to follow her home.

'Nice try but I need some sleep. And you, mister ...' She pressed my shirt, '... are trouble. Don't forget to call.'

Halfway through the night, Mandy had left with the Incredible Hulk, but I was happy to lose myself in Lucy. Now, with the orange glow of the highveld sun skirting the horizon, I felt the bile in my mouth, along with the ashy dryness of too many cigarettes. While driving everyone home, a thought popped into my head.

'Hey guys, fancy some ice cream?'

Unanimous choruses of approval rang out. 'I could *smash* a Cornetto!' shouted Kobus. Even Angela, who was typically reserved, let out an enthusiastic yelp.

And so it was that after a big night out, the bedraggled interns of the Jackson firm found themselves sitting on a car bonnet on Munro Drive, watching the sunrise, ice creams in hand, discussing life.

'Would you rather take on a horse-sized duck or a duck-sized horse?' Kobus giggled as he asked.

'The duck-sized horse any day of the week! What's it going to do, nip you? The horse-sized duck on the other hand ... that sounds freaky! Have you *seen* the ducks at Zoo Lake attack the bread?' Anwar was laughing uncontrollably. I was basking in the good vibes and decided it was time to take a risk.

'Hey guys,' I said. 'I have something to tell you. The reason I volunteered to drive tonight was because I wanted you all to have a good time ... but also ... I'm a recovering alcoholic. So, there's that.' I licked the chocolate crusting on my cone self-consciously. 'It's something I try not to be ashamed of, but I still am sometimes. But you seem like good people and I wanted you to know. I didn't want to have to lie every time you offered me a drink. It also keeps me accountable, you know? Now I can't drink in front of you and pretend like that's a normal thing.'

'Hey man, my uncle has the same problem except he still drinks. It really fucks good people up. I'm happy for you,' Kobus responded kindly.

'Ja, that's awesome. Just let us know if you need anything,' Angela said.

'I'm good. It's been quite a while, but sometimes I still get the cravings. Ice cream helps, so ... if you're ever worried, then you have to buy me ice cream. Immediately. Only Magnums count. Preferably almond.'

'On our salaries? Forget it. You're getting the local soft serve from that dodgy dude outside the hospital and that's *it*,' said Anwar.

'Deal!'

'Well cheers to ice cream then!' shouted Kobus.

'Cheers!' we all said in unison. It had been a while since I had been part of a team. We weren't exactly The Avengers, but whatever we were was a hell of a lot better than facing Bara alone.

We finished our ice creams and I then dropped everyone off. I crashed out as soon as I got home. It felt so good for the ache in my body to be from something other than the hospital.

I awoke a few hours later in a thick sweat. Although I had the rest of the weekend off, I couldn't stop thinking about the work I hadn't managed to finish during the week. The X-rays I hadn't had time to review, the sputum samples I hadn't been able to collect, the blood culture results that were pending. I knew that while there was ward call over the weekend, they were only there for urgent, potentially life-threatening issues, not to pick up my slack.

I tried to watch a movie on TV but thoughts kept invading my brain. What if? What if you sit here and the X-ray shows a type of pneumonia you aren't covering? What if the patient has TB and it's getting worse because you couldn't send the sample off in time? What if the blood culture shows a bacteria that is life-threatening?

I remembered Phelo's words about not doing unnecessary additional work, but my body was already moving. Cursing myself, I changed into casual clothes and drove to Bara. The music I was listening to in my car was bland indie rock and in the song the lead singer compared his girlfriend to hot chocolate lemonade. Previously, this song had delighted me, but the earnest melodies and witty wordplay grated and felt a million miles away from the gritty hospital and impoverished patients I was going to see. What the hell is a hot chocolate lemonade, anyway?

I turned the stereo off and listened to the silent road beneath my car. Thunder rumbled in the distance and I could see dark clouds looming.

When I entered the ward, I quickly reviewed the patients and gave Mr Mbalathi (who we thought might have TB) a small container, which I asked him to cough into, hoping to send some sputum to the lab for analysis. I told Sister Ndlovu to monitor him and call me when we had something. I had barely been gone five minutes when I heard her admonishing voice.

'Hawu! Buthi! What is this?' I walked to Mr Mbalathi's bed. In the specimen container was a large worm which he had just hacked up. It was wriggling and writhing. I recognised it as *Ascaris lumbricoides*, a worm that lives in the intestine of someone who has swallowed one of its eggs, prevalent in the soil in South Africa. Usually, it doesn't cause too many problems, but Mr Mbalathi had generated so much pressure in his abdomen trying to cough for us that the worm had been expelled.

'What are we supposed to with this?' she said sternly, without missing a beat. 'Test the *worm* for TB?' She shook her head. 'Try again.'

Eventually, she emerged with a small container full of sputum. This was great, but I needed three separate specimens, and Mr Mbalathi had fallen fast asleep. I didn't have the heart to wake him up. Looking again, I could see that there was enough sputum in the container I was holding to divide into two more. I sourced an N95 mask, some gloves from the nurses' station and walked to the sink.

Sputum is thick and doesn't pour easily. I had to scoop the contents out with my hands and pull the mucousy mix apart. It reminded me of play dough except it smelled terrible and was probably crawling with TB bacteria. After handling the gelatinous goop, I took another container, which I needed for Ms Khumalo who had developed diarrhoea. I went to her bed, undid the nappy covering her pelvis, and scooped some of the loose stool into the plastic container.

Almost every doctor has their kryptonite – a type of bodily fluid they hate. For some it's vomit; for others, urine or lung sputum. Mine was (and remains) faeces. I found the smell overpowering and my eyes watered as I ladled the loose stools with a wooden tongue depressor. I thought back to the early days of med school and how I had something slightly more glamorous in mind when I thought about internship life.

The only good thing about being at the hospital on my weekend off was that I had something to distract me from thoughts of Mandy. It also gave me an excuse not to return Lucy's texts. They had been friendly enough, but it was clear I would have some navigating to do during the week.

The storm clouds I had seen driving in suddenly burst and water engulfed the hospital. The corrugated roofs shuddered and leaks sprang everywhere, including above Mr Mbalathi's bed. We moved

PART 1: THE PRESENTATION

him a foot to the right and placed a bucket under the dripping water. Despite the noisiness, the dense rain cleared the air of dust and grime. When I walked to my car four hours later there was a unique freshness in the air, with crickets chirruping happily.

On a whim, I decided to check on the marijuana field. It was drowning in a puddle of muddy, oil-shiny water. The rain had hit the rock-hard earth and formed a deluge rather than being absorbed into the ground. There was a foul odour and mosquitoes were already accumulating.

I was no gardener but even I could tell that garden was in trouble. Prof Waters would have his work cut out trying to save it.

I retraced my steps and drove home.

Chapter 4
ON THE CLOCK

'You don't change Baragwanath; Baragwanath changes you.' Someone had tacked a piece of paper with this unattributed quote onto the office pinboard. It was old and faded, but its enduring presence on a board that was adjusted daily spoke to the reverence with which many regarded its advice.

I realised after a few weeks at Bara that something needed to change. Staying afloat on the sea of patients was becoming harder and harder. I didn't have the self-belief yet to confidently discharge patients and Chloe seemed distracted, often disappearing for entire afternoons to see her research supervisor or to attend to personal matters.

When we entered yet another intake day with thirty-two patients still on our list, an exasperated Chloe had had enough. 'Do you *ever* discharge anyone?'

I was also doing my best to avoid Lucy, whose texts I had surreptitiously deleted without a response after our night together. The longer I left the situation, the more awkward I knew an explanation would be, which made me ignore it even longer. If I saw her walking down a corridor, I ducked into the nearest ward, pretending to be doing something important. Once, she phoned me to turf back a patient and I had accepted and hung up without even getting their details. Phelo took particular delight in my predicament, sometimes falsely screeching that he could see her coming and laughing hysterically when I ducked under a nurse's desk or into a storage closet.

When I wasn't doing my best to remain incognito, I was trying to reason my way out of my expanding list of patients. The maths was simple and I had always been good at maths. If I had forty-five patients to get through, and I spent on average seven minutes per patient (five seeing them, one making notes, one walking to the next bed), then working through the inpatients would take me five hours and fifteen minutes. This was the best-case scenario and didn't take into account the additional time that a sick or deteriorating patient would need, how long additional procedures took, or questions that occasionally arose when Chloe or Prof Waters popped in.

So the best-case scenario was: arrive at 7am, collect results until 8am, see patients until 1:15pm. This left me just under four hours for consults, discharges, procedures, family discussions, radiology requests, nursing queries and other updates.

This was manageable (just) but it would require discipline not to deviate. Even an extra minute per patient could put me an hour behind in the afternoon.

Given these small slots of time for each patient, I no longer had the luxury to enquire about anything except the illness that had brought the patient to hospital. Listening to Phelo's advice about focusing on one problem only, I learned to stop vaguely asking patients how they were feeling as this could take over four minutes of our precious time. (I quickly learned that for some patients talking about their maladies was a form of nostalgia.)

'Well, Doctor, where can I begin? My knee pain from the soccer injury I got a few years ago is acting up. It always does in the cold and the nurses leave the windows open at night – this ward is freezing! My chest is a bit better but the sputum has gone from yellow to brown and I'm not sure if that's a good thing? Could it be the cigarettes? The prongs from the oxygen are hurting my nose – I broke it a few years ago when a tsotsi tried to rob me – and I was wondering if you could perhaps get smaller ones? I'm also a bit worried about the rat I saw running outside. I've always had a fear of rats ...'

From now on, I would keep things focused and direct.

'How are the lungs today, Mr Radebe?'

'Is your leg feeling better, Ms Kuzwayo?'

'Any rash from the TB drugs, Mr Mbayi?'

When patients tried to expand upon their illnesses, I politely shepherded them back to the original complaint. Sometimes, I had to be firmer.

'Where is the pain the *worst*, sir?'

'Well, Doctor ... it hurts here. But it also hurts here. And I have a pretty dreadful headache. And I'm coughing. And I felt a bit nauseous after my food last night. And ...'

'Okay, okay. Which of those would you say is the *biggest* problem for you today?'

'Doctor, they're all pretty big.'

'But if you could choose one?'

'I suppose ... the headache?'

'Fine. I'll write up some Panado. That should make you feel better.'

'Oh, and Doc? My family is coming round this afternoon. They'd like to talk to you. Could you come?'

'I'll see. It's clinic, so no promises.' Already I was checking my watch. I had spent too much time on Mr Radebe.

'Oh, and Doc ...?'

But I was already on my way out the ward. 'One problem at a time, Mr Radebe!'

Clinic was an opportunity to follow up on patients Chloe and I had discharged; to see how they were doing. We also inherited the patients our predecessors in earlier blocks had been managing. That afternoon the first person through the door was Ms Jacobs, from my first ever intake. Seeing her name again was startling. Chloe and I had discharged her after her lung abscess had responded well to two weeks of IV therapy. In addition to prescribing a few weeks' worth of oral antibiotics, I had made some adjustments to her insulin, and started her on a tablet for her blood pressure. I was really hoping that we'd see an improvement so when the nurse handed me a slip of paper with the results, the disappointment stung.

Her readings were, if possible, even worse than they had been prior to discharge. I was shocked. How was this even possible? Had I made a mistake with her medication? The shock soon gave way to irritation. Ms Jacobs was supposed to represent a win for me – she should have been much better by now. We should have been celebrating an improvement in her health. Now I would have to spend even more time trying to get to the bottom of what was wrong, and an imposingly large group of patients was still waiting to be seen.

She shuffled in and I immediately began interrogating her. Was she taking the medication? Yes, Doctor. Was she getting enough sleep? Yes, Doctor. Was she taking her antibiotics? Yes, Doctor. Was she eating right? Yes, Doctor. Are you sure?

She faltered and I saw an opening. 'Ms Jacobs?'

'Well, you see, Doctor. It was my late husband's birthday last week. He *loved* chocolate cake. Especially the way I make it, so ... I made one for him because remembering him happy makes me happy. But there was no one to share it with. The kids are too old for silly things like eating cake with their mother. So ... I just had it all myself.' She bowed her head and a single tear slid down her cheek. 'I'm sorry. I know you said I should avoid too much sugar but what else was I supposed to do with it? I was sad and it made me feel better. I couldn't just throw it away.'

'Ms Jacobs, I understand. I know how you feel ...'

She looked up. 'Do you? Do you really? Have you lost a husband or wife? Someone you shared your life and dreams with?'

I shifted uncomfortably. My attempt at empathy had fallen horribly flat and I had managed to make my patient feel even worse.

'Okay, let's begin again. Let's discuss your diet and exercise ...'

By the time I was finished with Ms Jacobs, an hour had whizzed by. We had managed to identify some troublesome foods that she agreed to cut down on, and we had forged a mini-exercise plan. We also made some minor adjustments to her meds based on the side effects. ('The water tablet makes me pee all through the night, Doctor. I don't like it.') The plan we came up with was by no means perfect, but we had created it together and she seemed a lot happier. When I ushered her out, I felt the glow of having made a difference.

The glow was short-lived though when I saw the grumpy patients waiting to see me. They had been waiting for hours and there were taxis they needed to catch to get home. The bottom line was that as much as I wanted to spend time with each of them, getting to the core of their problems, there just weren't enough hours in the afternoon. I hurried through, doing the best I could, but by the time I shuffled out, I was exhausted and still had patients in the ward to sort out. Ms Jacobs was a win ... but was it a Pyrrhic victory? As a result of all the time I had spent with her, I had little left for the rest of the clinic, and I had to rush through without any meaningful engagement. Would I have been better off trying to carve the time out equally? Ms Jacobs had seemed so distressed that cutting her short would have been unkind. But having to rush everyone else was cruel and unfair, too. I had no idea how to balance the needs of my individual patients against the needs of the entire list, especially when time was so limited. What if the grumpy ones felt it was no longer worth their while to wait so long and never came back? Could I blame them? The patience shown by people at Baragwanath often bordered on the saintly, but everyone has their limit. Was I pushing people over theirs? I puzzled over this dilemma as I made my way back to the ward.

I only managed to leave work at 11pm that night and was so tired I almost didn't notice the long line of women shuffling in front of my car until I nearly drove into them. I slammed on brakes, but they barely seemed to notice. Many were coughing, some were carrying IV bags attached to their arms, the transparent connecting tubes filled with blood flowing backwards from their arms. I wondered for a moment, if in my exhausted state I was hallucinating, so strange was the sight. In a few minutes the women shuffled off and it was as if the hospital let out a sigh and swallowed the women into the darkness.

The next day workmen arrived and suddenly started installing blue lights into the ceilings in the wards. When I asked what was going on, Phelo said, 'UV lights. To kill TB.'

'Really?' I responded. 'Those are going to make the wards safer?' The lights were tiny and housed within a plastic contraption that looked like a fire alarm. The idea was that air would be filtered through them and the UV would kill the hardy mycobacteria floating around. Great idea in theory, but the ward was massive and there were only three lights throughout. It felt ... inadequate.

'These lights do absolutely nothing,' Prof Waters' voice echoed behind me. 'Come ... check it out.' He held a R100 note next to one of them. I wasn't sure what I was supposed to be looking at. The note appeared normal, albeit brightly lit.

'If this was proper UV we should see the watermark. But there's nothing. So ... this is just funky blue light giving us a gentle tan. Oh, and it's making someone rich. Hello sir!' He gesticulated to the foreman in the ward, 'How much do these peculiar devices cost?'

'About R20 000 each.'

Prof gave a low whistle. 'So if each ward has three, and there forty-six wards in this hospital, that's nearly a million bucks ... on funky blue lights that don't do anything. Niiiiiiice ...' He turned to me. 'So, how are our patients? Did I tell you that I came up with a collective noun for interns ...?'

Later that morning, I found Sister Ndlovu. I asked her about what I had seen the previous night and why sick women were trudging between the wards late at night.

'To make space,' she said perfunctorily.

'Space for what?'

'Well, during intake, you young doctors often admit everybody. You don't think about space.' She clucked her tongue against her teeth. 'So, to make room, we have to move people around.' She explained that when the ward was full, but more beds were needed, the healthier patients would be moved to other wards where there was space. This dance of musical chairs would be reversed a few days later when the ward they were in needed those beds back for their own intake. The patients would then be shuffled back or sent somewhere else with open beds.

'Who decides which patients move?' I asked.

'We do.'

'Oh. Why not the doctors?'

'Whenever we call you, you tell us you're too busy.'

'Why do they have to walk? Couldn't we get porters to move them?'

'Dokotela, where have you been? The porters are all busy in Ward 30. There are too many patients for them to keep up.'

'And why do we do this in the middle of the night when it's cold and dark?'

Sister Ndlovu gave me an unreadable look and shuffled off.

Later that day, a nurse I didn't know sidled up to me as I was passing the orthopaedic ward.

'Excuse me, but can you come inside?' she said. I was perplexed; I didn't have any patients in the ortho ward, so I assumed she had confused me for one of the surgeons.

'It's about Mr Mtombini.'

My heart stopped. It was the gentleman from my first day who had overdosed. After that post-call morning, during which I had been unable to find him, I had been so overwhelmed that he had fallen off my list. Since then, no one had alerted me to where he was so there had been no prompts to locate him. Now, it seemed, he had been situated in a random orthopaedic ward for weeks.

'He saw you walk past and said, "There's my doctor! I haven't seen him in a while!" so I thought I would call you,' she explained.

Mr Mtombini's statement that it had been 'a while' was euphemistic. It had been many weeks since that first day.

With my head bowed, and my heart heavy, I followed her into the ward. This was a disaster. How could I have neglected a patient for so long? This feeling of guilt was followed by a brief spurt of anger. My name was on his admission notes so why had no one called me?

As I approached his bed, I saw him sitting up, chatting to a few of his neighbours in the ward, and laughing loudly. 'There he is! My doctor!'

'Mr Mtombini. I'm so dreadfully sorry I haven't ...' He cut me off with a wave of his hand.

'I've been very happy here. No point in you worrying about me.'

I grabbed his file at the foot of his bed, the tatty, well-thumbed document heavy in my hands. Other than the admission note from weeks ago, in the time he had been in the hospital, he had only been seen once, by the ward call intern when he was feeling nauseous and had a fever. He had originally been in the ophthalmology ward, before being moved to general surgery, then the Hendricks male ward, and then back to ophthalmology, before winding up in orthopaedics, where he had been for the past six days. All his medications had been dutifully given, and an antibiotic had been started when he had the fever. This antibiotic, which should only have been administered for a few days, was now on its third week and still being given to him religiously by the nurses.

The good news was that he appeared well so I told him that he could go home.

'Do I have to, Dokotela? I like it here ...'

'Yes, sir. We need the bed. Now, because of the overdose I want you to see the psychiatrists. I think you would perhaps benefit from some anti-depressant medications? Maybe someone to talk to?' Again, he waved me away.

'I've done this before, I know how it works. They'll only be able to see me in a year, maybe longer, and then maybe once or twice before they try to put me on pills. I don't like them. They make it hard for me to fulfil my duties. You know ...' He glanced down at his crotch.

I knew that some of the anti-depressants we prescribed could

PART 1: THE PRESENTATION

diminish libido. I had experienced that myself a few years before so I was sympathetic. Nevertheless, there was no longer any justification for keeping Mr Mtombini in hospital. He took it with good grace.

'You know, Dokotela. This place. It isn't so bad. Sometimes people do get better.'

I was dreading the moment I would have to tell Chloe about Mr Mtombini. How do you explain that you lost a patient for weeks on end? I consoled myself that it could have been worse. Kobus had had a particularly ill patient during one intake who was admitted with very little hope of surviving the night. The following morning, before the post-intake round, the patient's bed had curtains drawn around it, and Kobus had assumed the worst. He scratched the name off his list and continued his rounds. The next day, the patient's family wanted a quick word. They informed Kobus that, through the patient's sister, he was entitled to private medical aid. They wanted him transferred to a private hospital that evening. Kobus gathered his thoughts and informed the family that sadly the patient had passed away. He was dreadfully sorry, but he had arrived so unwell that there was little that could be done.

The family were confused. He was very much alive, they said, and they wanted him to be transferred. Kobus responded kindly that denial was part of the grieving process, that what they were experiencing was normal, but that unfortunately we couldn't undo the past. The family looked at him as if he were mad and reiterated their request. At that moment, Kobus heard a voice ring out, 'Doctor Kobus! I'm not dead!' It was the patient, sitting up and eating soup, appearing to be in vibrant health. The curtains had simply been drawn around his bed while he was having an impromptu bath. No one could decide if this was the best or worst healthcare in the world.

I decided to rip the band-aid off, so to speak, and tell Chloe rather than drag it out.

Weirdly, after hearing the story, she wasn't particularly fazed. For the past few days she had been distant and disengaged, and she muttered something about 'these things happening' before disappearing off.

Later that afternoon she was about to prescribe an antibiotic for a patient I knew they were severely allergic to. I stopped her just in time, but she was distraught at the near miss.

'I could've killed someone. I'm such a fool,' she said. I had never seen Chloe like this. She was always a model of consistency and reliability. When all else failed, Chloe would know what to do. Chloe *always* knew what to do. In my lower moments, I wondered if I would ever be as competent and knowledgeable as she was. Yet here she was, berating herself and doubting her own judgement.

'It's no biggie,' I said. 'You've saved my hide so many times it's about time I repaid the favour. I think the score is now Chloe 1432, Alastair 1.' My attempt at levity got a weak smile. I decided to press on.

'Chloe ... is everything okay? It's none of my business, but you seem a bit ... distracted today. Anything going on?'

'I'm just tired, is all. We have a busy list because you never discharge anyone!' She jokingly punched my shoulder. As I recoiled in mock pain, I saw her glance over my shoulder. The colour drained from her face and her whole body deflated. She spun around. Confused, I looked back. Walking towards us, with the practised intimacy of an established couple, was Dr Simpson and his wife.

They walked past us and Dr Simpson offered us the briefest of smiles. Chloe looked resolutely down at the concrete floor. Once they had gone past I said to her, 'Wanna grab a coffee?'

PART 1: THE PRESENTATION

It had been going on for months. What started as a legitimate research pairing had slowly blossomed over time into a full-blown romance.

'God, I'm such a cliché,' Chloe muttered. 'I knew his reputation. But there's something about his passion for his patients. Before I knew it, we were staying late and discussing our life stories. He's miserable but he stays with her because if they split, she'll take the kids. When, one night, he put his hand on my thigh, I was so relieved. I'd been waiting so long and now it was finally happening ...'

At first, he promised Chloe he would leave his wife. But as time passed he had softened until, a few days before, he had broken it off with Chloe, citing the welfare of his children.

'Tale as old as time,' Chloe reiterated.

I wasn't sure where to train my eyes as I felt slightly uneasy at this level of 'closeness' between us. We were in the lone doctors' cafeteria at Baragwanath. It was a single room located in a central building close to the medical wards. It served the usual smorgasbord of fried, unhealthy food and greasy lunches. The coffee was usually burnt, but it was jam-packed with caffeine, and that was all that mattered. Looking back at Chloe, I didn't know what to say. She and Dr Simpson were both consenting adults; this sort of thing happened all the time. But it was clear Chloe didn't regard him as an equal; she held him in awe. The way she spoke about him reminded me of how kids refer to superheroes. It all felt ... icky. I couldn't think of a better word, but I couldn't say that to her in that moment.

'Chloe? Do you want to escalate this? There are rules about mentors having relationships with their mentees.'

'What good would that do? It's not like he'll come back to me. His marriage might end and the hospital will probably give him a slap on the wrist. I, on the other hand, will be known as the reg who slept with a married man and then tried to wreck his home life. It will be so embarrassing, I don't know if I'd ever live it down. No ... this one I think I'll keep to myself ... And please, whatever you do, promise me you won't tell anyone.'

'Chloe, I promise. If you don't want me to, I won't say a word to anyone.'

'Thank you.' She stared into her cup of coffee. 'You must think I'm an awful person.'

'I don't think that at all. I'm just worried about you, is all.'

'I'm fine. Don't worry about me.' I raised an eyebrow.

'Okay fine,' she laughed – for only the second time that day. 'I'll let you know if I'm not coping. I know you struggled at the beginning but you're a lot better these days.'

When we parted ways, nothing had been solved but the air between us felt clearer.

Chapter 5
COMRADES

It started as a murmur, but gradually, as the days went by, it got louder and louder until it drowned out all other conversation. An unthinkable idea that seemed more and more inevitable as time went on. Then it all blew up with a single notice on the staff board. STRIKE ACTION! SAVE OUR HOSPITAL! EMERGENCY MEETING FOR ALL PHYSICIANS AT 2PM IN THE OPHTHALMOLOGY AUDITORIUM.

There was a clucking behind me. Two patients on crutches were reading the announcement over my shoulder.

'Hawu! How can doctors go on strike? Madness! Who will look after us?!'

I wasn't sure if they knew I was a physician or not, so I decided to stay where I was rather than turning to face them.

'Doctors are pretty useless, my bra,' said the man next to him. 'They spend five seconds in the wards and then go back to their fancy offices. If the *nurses* go on strike ... we'd be fucked.'

In fact, a few years before when I was still in high school, the nurses *had* gone on a sudden, wild-cat strike. Baragwanath had been crippled; clinics had shut, wards had been abandoned, patients were turned away; some died. The hospital still bore the scars and stories of the time occasionally circulated. I once heard Anwar mutter, 'That nurse seems lovely now but during the strike, I heard she was part of the mob pulling ambulances over and hauling patients out.' I never did find out if that was true.

Resentments lingered like ash in the air. Nurses felt the doctors hadn't supported them; doctors felt nurses had gone too far and put patients needlessly at risk. A divide between the two had opened up.

No one, however, could remember doctors ever striking. Mere discussion of the topic was unprecedented. The chatter among the interns was rapid and intense. Doctors, we knew, were designated under law as 'essential labour', meaning we were not allowed to strike under any circumstances. As trainees, we were at particular risk because we needed the hospital to sign off our logbooks to enable us to meet the requirements of internship. Without this approval, we could not advance our careers.

There was also a deeper, more primal fear. We knew, deep down, that unlike some of the consultants, we were disposable. Specialist physicians were in short supply, and while the hospital essentially ran on the labour of interns, there were so many around that no one in management would worry too much about firing a few of us.

Over cigarettes, next to the marijuana field, the discussion among our group about whether to attend the meeting or not was fevered.

'Come on, let's just hear the people out,' Anwar said. 'It's not like we're committing to anything drastic.'

'... yet,' Phelo interjected. He let that linger before continuing. 'But by going aren't we admitting that it's at least a *possibility*? What does that say about us? That abandoning our patients if our demands aren't met is something we'd consider?'

PART 1: THE PRESENTATION

Angela was biting her lip worriedly. 'Is this meeting even sanctioned? Could we get into trouble just for going? What if management sends spies?'

'Don't be ridiculous,' Anwar scoffed. 'Doctors are allowed to meet and discuss shit, right?'

There was a sudden pause as we all thought the same thing. Earlier in the year, in response to growing calls for her to step down, the CEO of Baragwanath had issued an unofficial proclamation: doctors were not permitted to congregate in groups of more than five unless for strict academic purposes. Staff had obviously ignored such a ridiculous edict. One morning, a group of ten concerned surgeons had met to discuss issues affecting the hospital. They had debated going to the press. Someone must have ratted them out because word leaked to top management. Two surgeons were subsequently suspended for a week and were facing disciplinary hearings and the possibility of dismissal. Pleas in their defence had been resolutely ignored by management. It had been a sobering reminder of the capriciousness (but also the viciousness) with which the hospital defended its reputation.

'I'm going,' I said. 'There will be too many of us there for them to suspend us all. And we need to stand up for ourselves. Or are we just going to turn a blind eye to everything that goes on around us?'

'Hang on,' Phelo again interjected. 'Is this about the hospital? Or about our pay? They're separate issues and we should be clear.'

Feet scuffled.

'Couldn't it be both?' Anwar eventually said. 'We're part of this whole bloody system. We're massively underpaid. If doctors are unhappy and burnt out what happens in the rest of the hospital doesn't really matter. We can't keep propping things up.'

'But doesn't *everyone* feel that way?' Angela said. 'The registrars certainly do. The nurses earn, what, like, thirty bucks an hour or something. No consultant working in public service can send their kids to a good school. We're not unique.'

'They're building that fancy new emergency area,' Anwar responded. 'If they've got the millions for that they can spare a bit extra for the interns. How are we supposed to live on R8 000 a month?'

'Fine,' Phelo said. 'Let's hear them out. But strength in numbers, okay? We all go?' Heads nodded before heading back to work.

We knew walking into the meeting that things were likely to get heated. It started off uncontroversially enough. The nominated head of the registrars stood up and noted that we had reached a crossroads. Conditions were poor and patients were suffering. As an example, he brought up the CT scanner bookings. At the beginning of the previous year, they had been able to book outpatient CT scans for the patients who needed them. By the middle of the year, the waitlist had extended well into winter of the *following* year. This was exacerbated by one of the two scanners breaking down, and the maintenance company refusing to fix it because of unpaid bills owed to them by the hospital. In response, the radiology department had suddenly, and without warning, cancelled *all* CT outpatient scans, leaving hundreds in the lurch.

My patient, Ms Jacobs, had deteriorated over the past few months and I had booked a repeat scan to make sure the abscess in her lungs that we had treated hadn't returned. Having waited patiently for two months, she was one week away from her appointment when she received a terse phone call informing her that due to 'technical difficulties' her scan had been postponed indefinitely.

I had felt powerless and distraught in the face of her anger and disappointment. No amount of cajoling and pleading with radiology could change their minds. 'Rebook her and we'll see what we can do. Current wait time: seven months.' I could have readmitted her, as getting an inpatient scan was much less trouble, but she flat-out refused. 'I nearly died the last time I was here, Doctor. I can't go through that again.'

We had to come up with a contingency plan that neither I nor Ms Jacobs really bought into. And she was one of many.

Frequently, junior doctors were the face of a failing system, and it eroded our souls.

The head registrar's loud voice brought me back to the meeting. All but the hardiest or most dedicated were leaving for better environments, he said, which placed an unreasonable burden on junior doctors. Complaints through all the usual channels had failed; management had no real interest or motivation in addressing these issues, which had been simmering for years and had now reached boiling point. He noted that the only time the hospital looked clean was when a VIP or politician was visiting. Suddenly new curtains appeared around beds, plants sprang up in previously drab wards, floors were scrubbed mercilessly throughout the night, light bulbs that had been out for weeks were miraculously replaced. Baragwanath could be made to appear healthy, but like an abscess that hasn't been drained, it was festering underneath.

The issue of remuneration loomed large. Everyone felt underpaid. Tied into the pleas for better working conditions was a demand for a fifteen per cent wage increase across the board.

When someone pointed out that there was a global financial crisis and that we were entering a recession, with little additional money available, there were loud grumbles and murmurings.

'They had enough for those stupid blue TB lights!' someone shouted.

'They had enough to give the nurses a large raise a few years ago!' grumbled another.

Phelo raised his hand. His history as an anti-apartheid activist in his school days lent him an air of immediate authority. 'Comrades. Let us be specific. What exactly are we talking about here? We just ... don't come to work ... or what? No services at all? Some services? We all know what happens to patients if we just stay home ...'

Someone leapt up. 'If we don't go all in and support each other the hospital will carry on and nothing will change.'

Phelo regained his authority. He calmly said, 'So I ask again: what does a strike for doctors look like? Don't forget – public support was with the nurses' strike until people started dying ...'

After some chatter, a proposal was put forward that emergency services should remain open but everything else should close. There was general nodding until one of the nephrology registrars raised her hand. 'We have to maintain dialysis services. Our programme keeps hundreds of people with kidney failure alive every week. And it's not like they'll just be okay without dialysis for a while. Every day matters.'

'And what about the wards?' Kobus chimed. 'If emergency services are open, then patients will be admitted. Who's going to look after them in the wards? And discharge the patients who are better to make way for the new ones?'

The senior registrar who opened the meeting held up his hand to restore order. 'So ... what I'm hearing is that emergency services, dialysis and wards will stay open. All clinics, however, will shut.'

At this point, the endocrinology registrar raised her hand. She murmured too softly at first, and a chorus resounded for her to speak up.

'I have patients on insulin.' Her voice was trembling. 'If our clinic closes they won't be able to get it. They'll either die or present to emergency in ketoacidosis. I know my patients and I'm not willing to do that to them. So I don't think that I, in good conscience, could close our clinic.' She sat down and stared at the floor.

A cardiologist then chimed in. 'We can't close ours either. Patients are on cardiac meds that are literally keeping them out of heart failure. We can't interrupt that.'

'Why not just keep them all on the same meds? The pharmacists aren't striking,' someone shouted.

'... yet ...' someone grumbled. There was nervous laughter.

'Can't we just have someone write all the prescriptions then? Maybe an intern? But that's *all* they do? No actual patient interactions?'

'We can't put this all on the interns. What happens when they get a dose wrong or something? They'd be medico-legally responsible.'

'So what's the bloody point of a strike then?' someone shouted in frustration. 'Emergency will be open, wards will be open, clinics will mostly be open ... it's like business as bloody usual!'

Everyone's phones beeped at once. Friends and colleagues from other hospitals had been sending us information all afternoon to keep us updated. This sudden and coordinated chorus suggested, however, that something big had just happened.

An uneasy silence filled the room. One of the orthopaedic interns stood up. 'Tembisa Hospital has gone on a full strike! All services shut!' There were gasps and some smatterings of applause. It was real. This was happening.

'We have to join them,' he continued. 'Now's the time!'

'Can't we just hang on a bit and talk this through?' Phelo pleaded.

'No! If all other hospitals strike and we're the only one working ... where do you think all the patients will go?' The words settled on us like a heavy blanket.

The air in the room was becoming thick and clogged. The sense that this was all spiralling rapidly out of control was palpable, yet a decision had to made.

Suddenly, the auditorium door slammed open and a short woman, flanked by two tall, muscular men, strode purposefully to the front. I knew immediately who it was even though I'd never met her. The CEO. Her composure and comportment were stern; it was clear that she was not coming as an ally.

There was a palpable shift in the energy of the room. Her presence cast sudden doubt on the legitimacy of our meeting and, for a moment, we felt like naughty schoolchildren awaiting a scolding from the headmistress.

Without being asked, she took to the podium, glanced around, cleared her throat and then spoke forcefully into the microphone.

'Comrades,' she began, 'we have heard that there are talks about possible strike action at Baragwanath. In case you have forgotten, a reminder ...' She paused for emphasis. 'You. Are. Essential. Workers ...' Her long, blood-red, perfectly manicured talon-like nails jabbed the podium after each word, '... and you *cannot strike*. Management will take any – and all! – disciplinary steps against any doctor who is not working at one hundred per cent capacity. Employees in violation of this will face dismissal. Trainees and interns, if you participate you will *not* be signed off. We've faced this sort of nonsense from you people before and we were victorious. Please don't test our resolve.' She let that comment linger before continuing. 'I'm sure you are aware that other hospitals in Gauteng have begun unsanctioned strike action. Rest assured, I have been in contact with the minister and the CEOs. It's just a small minority of disruptive agents and they will be dealt with. Trying to emulate them would be ... a mistake.'

She paused, slowly removed a handkerchief from her handbag, and patted beads of sweat from her forehead.

PART 1: THE PRESENTATION

'I understand you have grievances. We all know this hospital has challenges. But this is unacceptable. Un. Ac. Ceptable. The health minister and I are in accordance about working conditions and he assures me that extra funds are being allocated as we speak. I have also spoken to His Excellency, President Zuma,' her voice swelled, 'and His Excellency has graciously informed me that he has looked at the numbers and while senior doctors are well compensated, junior doctors are earning too little. You will be getting a raise this year; the exact sum to be determined. But it will not be insignificant.'

Phelo leaned over to me and whispered, 'Divide and conquer. Oldest trick in the book ...'

The CEO continued, 'Now ... I have been hearing rumours of doctors speaking to the press. I want to remind you that you signed a contract. And that contract prohibits disclosing hospital matters to journalists without the express approval of human resources.

'The press, comrades, are not your friends. They will twist your words and do anything to make this hospital look bad. They've had an agenda for years.'

'Excuse me, Madam CEO,' the head registrar politely interjected, the fire in his voice nearly completely extinguished. 'I agree about the press, but our contracts *do* permit protest action. If you'll just see hospital guidelines, section 3, subsection b–'

'Yes, yes. Thank you for reminding me, comrade.' She swatted his comment away like an insect. 'Which brings me to my next point. Hospital management respects your rights. Many of us liberated this country through successful protest. If you still wish to go ahead, management will permit you to march through the hospital and around the periphery ... but only during your lunch hour. No patient care can be compromised and hospital security will be escorting you.' She paused. 'But remember what we did to traitors and tsotsis during the struggle ...' For the first and only time during that meeting, a smile traced across her lips. With that she hopped off the podium and marched back to her office.

True to their word, a few days later, the government increased the salaries of junior doctors substantially. This took the sting out of the hospital march, which was scheduled to take place a week later. Many interns felt their demands had been met and dropped out of further protest. Others felt there was more to our action than simply plumping our salaries – that we were protesting for a higher purpose and improved patient care. Many of the senior doctors were too burnt out and disheartened to participate. Prof Waters smiled wanly when I told him what our plan was. 'You cannot change this hospital, lad. I've seen it tried many times before and it never works.'

Nevertheless, on a rainy and cold weekday afternoon, a motley group of physicians assembled at one side of the hospital. Made up of senior consultants all the way to medical students, we marched resolutely through the corridors, our voices clanging and reverberating off the corrugated iron. A few bored-looking journalists had assembled, taking pictures intermittently, but the overall interest from the outside world was minimal. When we realised that only those in the wards were paying any attention to our chanting and singing (a furious nurse had berated us: 'You are making too much noise! We are trying to nap!'), we took the protest outside hospital grounds. As we marched down Klipfontein Road there were some half-hearted cheers from passers-by, but mostly amusement at the fancy folk in white coats protesting. I remember hearing some giggles, too. When it was over, we all went back to work and had to try to frantically catch up as we almost always worked through our lunch hour anyway. I left Baragwanath that day after 10pm.

PART 1: THE PRESENTATION

For a while, it felt like no one had even noticed. Almost nothing appeared in the press and life as we knew it at Bara continued. But we were wrong. One group *had* been paying close attention: the porters. Inspired by our call to action, they decided to strike the following week. Unlike the doctors, they didn't dither over the decision. One day they were there and the next they were ... gone. Suddenly our patients were without transport to get around the massive arteries of Bara, and it was chaos. They couldn't go for their scans or tests; they couldn't be transferred from the emergency areas to the wards; they couldn't be taken for their surgeries. The nurses resolutely refused to push the wheelchairs, stating (reasonably) that porter duties were not in their job descriptions, and that their hands were already full with patient care.

We initially thought that this was an easily fixable problem. Surely just about any able-bodied person could be a porter? All it required was some strength and elbow grease. Finding replacements with so much unemployment in the country would surely be easy?

We were wrong. The complex labour laws governing the hospital, combined with ominous threats from some unions, meant that no one could be fired, and no one could be hired as temporary replacements. We quickly realised that we were on our own. The only solution was to push the patients ourselves.

There is a certain skill to being a porter at Baragwanath. The concrete passage floors are often angled, which causes all transport to list to one side. This wasn't helped by the numerous bumps and cracks in the flooring that made the journey tricky if you weren't aware of them, and downright hazardous if you were. The easiest objects to manoeuvre were wheelchairs, whereas the most difficult were the stretchers, especially if any of the wheels were broken or legs were faulty (which was frequently the case).

One night, Kobus and Anwar were wheeling a patient to a CT

scan to clear a potential neck fracture. Next to radiology, the floor shifted unexpectedly from a hard left incline to a hard right. They were already battling a broken wheel that made the stretcher unstable and difficult to shift. In the darkness, they didn't see the change in the floor angle until it was too late. The stretcher started sliding downwards towards the bushes. At this point, the patient woke up from their alcohol-induced stupor and panicked, lunging for something to hold onto, and in this case it was the string on Kobus's scrub pants. He was pulled off his feet onto the stretcher and the additional weight only hastened the velocity of the duo downhill, leaving Anwar frantically running after them. I was attending to a patient in the ward when I heard a yelp and a crash and rushed out to see two naked bottoms poking out of the foliage in the moonlight – the patient's (where his flimsy gown had opened), and Kobus's (where the force of the crash and the strength of the patient's grip had sheared his scrubs and underwear right off). There was cursing and groaning and a melee of flailing limbs. Eventually we managed to get the patient back on the stretcher but immediately noticed he was without his neck collar. This was always kept on until we knew the patient didn't have a fracture of the spinal bones in their neck. Losing it presented a major problem.

'Let's just get him to the scanner,' Anwar pleaded.

'Hang on a bit. I can't find my bloody shoe!' Kobus grumbled.

After a few minutes of scrabbling around, they realised they would find neither in the darkness and thick greenery and decided to return in a few hours when it was light.

When two interns, one covered in scratches and one without a shoe, pushed a man into the CT department for his scan, the radiologist took one look and said, 'You're the folks here with the patient for CT spine? But lemme guess? You came off there by

PART 1: THE PRESENTATION

the turn? You're the third this week. Did the patient crash off the stretcher?'

Anwar and Kobus nodded sheepishly.

'Better make it a CT head as well,' he said.

Chapter 6
THE PIT

'**D**OCTOR, YOU NEED TO COME.'

Sister Khumalo couldn't have picked a worse time to interrupt me. I was midway through my sixth suture, and it required all my concentration to get it right. The man had a jagged wound on his face that canyoned raggedly from his eyebrow to his jaw. The cause of this laceration was a broken bottle wielded by his jealous best friend, who was lying in the bed next to him a few feet away. The waft of cheap beer was mingled with self-pity as both men groaned and wailed.

'I'm sorry I hit you with the bottle, my bra, but I saw you looking in *that* way at Fatima. You know how jealous I sometimes get, mos.'

'And I'm sorry I stabbed you,' my patient gestured at the stitches in his friend's neck, which Kobus had had to stitch to close an artery that had been spurting blood metronomically around the room. 'But after you hit me, I just *lost* it. No one hits me and gets away with it.'

'Sir, I can't stitch if you talk. It moves all the muscles,' I admonished.

'Sorry, Doctor. I'm just explaining myself, mos.'

PART 1: THE PRESENTATION

The nurse spoke again. 'Alastair, you need to come *now*.'

Sister Khumalo was an old hand in The Pit (our name for trauma admissions). No one knew exactly how long she'd been there, and if you asked, she would smile knowingly and say, 'Too long. Far too long.' When she raised the alarm, however, we all listened.

I put down the instruments, apologised to the patient, and stepped outside. 'What's up?'

She gestured to a little old lady sitting quietly on the bench, waiting to be seen. She had been there for about an hour and I must have walked past her at least a dozen times without giving her a second glance. I looked at the tatty file on her lap and noted that she had been in a pedestrian vehicle accident ('PVA' as we called them) but was triaged as 'yellow', meaning that although she needed to be seen as quickly as possible, she was not regarded as urgent.

It was a Saturday night after a Kaizer Chiefs versus Orlando Pirates soccer match. A derby between the two biggest soccer teams in Soweto was always met with dread by the team covering The Pit. We knew, regardless of the result, that there would be heavy drinking from the supporters of both sides. Whenever there was heavy drinking in Soweto, the loose lid that barely contained the daily frustrations and resentments of a marginalised community was blown off. Trauma and injuries, we knew, would follow.

Tonight had been no different, and a relatively quiet afternoon had ruptured, like an inflamed appendix, into total carnage at around 9pm. The Pit, with its four high-care bays and six regular rooms, was quickly overwhelmed. Stretchers snaked along the corridors on both sides. Soon they could no longer be contained in the building and spilled out into the chilly night air of the Gauteng winter. The registrars were all in theatre doing their best to repair various broken bodies, which meant that The Pit was being manned entirely by four nurses, two medical officers and three interns. We were clearly in damage-control mode and any case triaged any colour other than red ('life-threatening injury, must be seen immediately') had to wait.

I approached the little old lady with Sister Khumalo.

'Hello, ma'am. What's the problem?'

Quietly, almost ashamedly, she opened her coat, revealing three neat patches of blood, one above her heart, the other two over her abdomen. The patches were fresh and expanded visibly in front of my eyes.

'Oh, holy shit!' The words escaped my mouth before I had time to think. 'Those are bullet wounds!' I grabbed the chart. 'I don't understand? It says here she was in a PVA not that she had been shot!'

'Well, they ran me over after they shot me,' she said. Her words were barely a whisper, as if she were the one who had done something wrong.

'Goddammit. Take her into the resus bay immediately!'

Sister Khumalo shook her head. 'Can't. It's full.'

'Well, get someone out!' I ran to the resus bays to see how they looked. The area was a flurry of red chaos. Two patients had sustained burns over fifty per cent of their bodies and were being frantically revived by Phelo. One guy had been shot in the head but, remarkably, was still conscious and singing a bawdy tavern song in full voice. Another had been beaten so badly he looked barely human – a case of vigilante justice after he had been accused of stealing a neighbour's car. None of these patients could be moved and there was no space for an additional bed. I ran back to my original room, where both men were curled up and snoring.

'We need to move them out.' I turned to one of the medical students and told her she could finish the suturing.

'I've never stitched a face before.' Her German accent quivered.

PART 1: THE PRESENTATION

A visitor from Berlin, Gerta had been with us for just four days. This elective block was turning out to be more than she bargained for. 'What if I do it badly?'

Sister Khumalo had no time for such prevaricating. 'Hawu, look at him! He's already ugly! Who cares if the stitches aren't straight!' And with that, two porters magically appeared and wheeled the men out.

The elderly lady was wheeled in on a stretcher and I started with my ABCs: Airway, Breathing, Circulation. Her airway was patent and she was speaking to me. This was a huge relief because we didn't have the equipment to intubate her. Her breathing was rapid, but she was oxygenating her blood reasonably well – the saturation monitor on her finger was showing a reassuring 95%. Sister Khumalo held an oxygen mask over her face and I listened to the patient's lungs. The one beneath the bullet hole was dull, which meant blood or air had probably seeped in and now surrounded the lung. I needed an X-ray to confirm.

Sister Khumalo quickly wrapped the cuff of the automated blood pressure machine around her arm, but after some confused beeps, the machine sighed exhaustedly and turned itself off. After we had established that it couldn't be revived, and no other automatic machines were available, I grabbed the cuff I kept in my bag and manually checked her pressure, trying to keep my hands steady as I inflated it by squeezing the rubber bulb. It was too large for her arm, but it was the only one we had so it would have to do. Fortunately, her pulses were strong and there was no evidence she had lost too much blood.

As per the protocol, I took two large-bore IV lines from the resus bay and searched for the biggest veins she had. The lines went in and I started running clear normal saline through them. A quick review of her abdomen didn't reveal anything immediately alarming, and neither of the entry holes (Were they entry holes? Or exit holes? Or both? Shit, I couldn't remember how to tell the difference. I cursed my brain that had retained the pointless organic chemistry from first year but had rapidly forgotten important stuff like this) were close to the liver or spleen. But it was impossible to know with certainty what was going on internally, and which organs had been damaged.

Suddenly, her oxygen saturations started to drop, and her breathing, which had been rapid but controlled, took on a laboured intensity. Shit. The blood or air around her lung was compressing it like a vice, inhibiting its ability to expand and fill with air. We needed to relieve the pressure. I ran back to a resus bay and grabbed a chest tube kit and some sterile gloves. I started cleaning her chest in preparation, located the important anatomical landmarks, made a small incision in the side of her chest between her ribs, and bluntly opened the cut with the forceps. I had to be careful not to push too hard or I could damage her lung. I was aiming to find the area between the lung and the chest wall – the 'pleural space'. The patient was thin and as there was little fat in her chest, the forceps moved easily and before long I felt a subtle 'give'. There was an audible 'whoosh' as air rushed out, followed by a gush of dark blood. I took the tube and inserted it into the hole, but not before I felt my feet drenched with blood. With the tube in place, the blood and air that had been compressing her lung was draining out, allowing her to breathe easier. The compressed lung was able to expand and the oxygen saturations in her blood increased. I sutured the drain to her skin as best I could, and then called the registrar who was in theatre. Seamus was an Irish guy from Dublin, at Bara on his elective, and he didn't mince his words.

'Sounds like she needs to come to theatre immediately for a surgical assessment of her abdomen,' he said. 'Let's get her along.'

PART 1: THE PRESENTATION

Thirty minutes later, with the assistance of a porter, I wheeled the patient past the groaning queue of stretchers, carefully dodging hanging limbs, and out into the fresh evening air. The trip was a few hundred metres, made more perilous by a broken wheel on the stretcher that caused it to list dangerously to starboard. Eventually we got her into theatre where the surgeons were waiting. I gave a brief explanation of what had happened and what I had done. Seamus's face remained unchanged and he looked at my notes, the lines in her arms, and her chest drain, with forensic scrutiny.

'Let's be honest, that wasn't a perfect resus was it? And your notes are a bit sparse.' His Irish lilt only seemed to sharpen the criticism.

'No, Seamus, I guess it wasn't. But it all happened so quickly that I didn't really have time to write everything down.'

'We'll discuss it tomorrow on handover.' And with that, I was dismissed.

Walking back to The Pit, I reflected how weird the sudden changes in the past few weeks had been. A few weeks before, I was still in my general medicine block, preparing for handover to the intern who would be taking over from me. I didn't know who they would be, or what they would think of the state of my patients, so I did my best to make my handover list as thorough as possible. Where tests or tasks were still outstanding, I tried apologetically to explain what the hold-up had been. I hoped that whoever they were they would show me grace and not roll their eyes at my failures or shortcomings. Critiquing another's work with the aid of time and retrospection was easy; putting yourself in their shoes when Ward 30 was heaving, time was short and the pressure was on, was much less so.

Saying farewell to my patients was much harder than I expected. Some of the newer ones, I suspected, would barely notice that a new intern had taken over their management. But some of the older ones certainly might. I knew I would miss high-fiving Mr Mtshali every time we got him out of a diabetic coma and he could go home. Mornings would be strange without Ms Johnson's insistence that we pray together before I move on. Her leathery hand tightly gripping mine, she always asked God to help *me*, never herself. Mr Okorafor and his disbelief that I wouldn't accept money for seeing him. Mrs Fortune and her tears of joy when I brought her the rusks she so craved. And finally, Ms Jacobs. On our final clinic, I glanced at her file. I had eventually managed to get the CT scan we needed, which showed complete resolution of her lung abscess. Her blood sugars were well controlled, her cholesterol reasonable. We weren't there yet (her blood pressure was still too high and depression around her husband's passing still reared its head), and my successor still had work to do, but we had come a long way from that first admission on my first day. She seemed genuinely sad when I told her this was goodbye.

'You know, people say this hospital is terrible. In many ways it is but you young doctors give me hope. We all get hope when we see how much you care under these conditions.' Then she handed me a box of home-made biscuits and gave me a warm hug.

Bara was not the best. But the patients, from their willingness to endure incredible waiting times, put up with poor facilities, navigate the often impenetrable bureaucracy, and still keep coming back with gratitude for the care they received, certainly were.

And then the next day I was doing surgery, more specifically trauma. Once again we were expected to hit the ground running and we were thrown into the thick of it. No orientation, no lectures, little by way of introduction. There were patients to be seen and we had to start seeing them. What little confidence I had built up in my medicine

PART 1: THE PRESENTATION

block was suddenly dashed. Once again, I felt overwhelmed and completely out of my depth. Confronting me was a totally different environment, with totally different patients, new consultants, new nurses, new colleagues. I felt a sympathy for the patients in the ward with whiplash. This pattern of being thrown into a new specialty just as I was beginning to get a handle on the existing one, was to become a regular and cruel feature of internship. But there was also an excitement, a feeling of a new beginning. Old mistakes could be set aside, souring relations could be abandoned, slates could be wiped clean. This was a chance to prove myself anew.

But back in The Pit, the rest of that evening flowed like treacle. We worked frantically to reduce the queue, but like a hydra every stretcher we cleared seemed to spawn two more in its place. At one point, ambulances were supposedly diverted away from Baragwanath for four hours to give us some breathing room. In reality, they just parked outside the gate until the diversion was declared over. As a result, the brief lull was followed by a terrible new onslaught of patients. Almost every one of them was either deeply intoxicated or had suffered an injury from someone who was. The smell of cheap beer and wine became, at times, overpowering.

At one point, a well-dressed white woman was wheeled in, and almost everyone stopped and stared because of how unusual a sight it was. People like her just didn't come to The Pit.

She had been mugged and stabbed in the wrist, but didn't have private medical aid, which was why she had landed up at Bara. The stab was deep and ugly, but hadn't hit any important nerves or blood vessels so she was triaged as orange, meaning she would probably only be seen sometime the next day by the next team. She was enraged.

'Honestly! I don't understand why I'm here! I'm not supposed to be here! I'm just *between* medical aids at the moment and there's that cool-off period. You know how it is. Please call my kids, they'll sort this out.' Eventually she became so loud that I had to try to pacify her. She was visibly relieved when she saw me.

'Oh good. Someone who understands me. This is a terrible mistake. I usually go to the private clinic in Milpark. If you call my kids, they'll get me back there.'

Unfortunately, it was the middle of the night and none of her children answered their phones. I reassured her that she would be okay until morning, when we would sort everything out. Her eyes welled with tears.

'Oh god. Oh *god*! This *place*! It's so … *awful*. How could anyone actually be treated here?' I looked around. Seen through her eyes, I understood what she meant. The walls with yellowing, shabby paint; the windows caked with dust; the smell of the antiseptic floor cleaner mingled with the sweat and odours of a hundred people crammed into a small space; the rumble of the heater competing in vain against the cold outside. I don't think this was anyone's idea of where they wanted to end up in the early hours of Sunday morning, but for most people in Soweto it was all they had.

Every day, handover took place in the trauma boardroom. Its hushed tones, oak table, comfy chairs and clean carpets were jarring when contrasted with the noisy chaos of The Pit. The twenty-four hours without a wink of sleep and barely any time to sit down had taken their toll on me. I was utterly exhausted and so hungry that even the deeply unappetising hospital food served to the patients looked tempting.

This meeting was the only thing that stood between me and being able to go home. Nevertheless, I was worried. The head of trauma was a small Russian man called Dr Petkov. A true leader in his field, he was deeply respected for his knowledge, but feared for his famously short temper, especially if his exacting standards were not met.

We ran through all the day's resuscitations and Anwar reported that he had managed a patient with a severe head injury who neurosurgery had not come to see. They had told him they would only intervene if the patient's level of consciousness improved. At this, Dr Petkov's fist slammed the desk so hard we all jumped.

"What? They said *what*?! That's like saying to a plant, "Tell you what. I'll give you water ... *if* you grow"! It's ridiculous! What was the name of the consultant?'

Anwar told him and before we could move, Dr Petkov whipped his phone out. He stormed out of the room and we could hear him shouting and cursing from next door. Five minutes later he returned, the vein on his forehead visibly bulging. 'The consultant will see the patient this morning. You were absolutely right to call. He will send you an apology shortly.' We all glanced at each other. A consultant defending an intern over a senior colleague? We had never witnessed anything like it.

Eventually, we got to the case of the old lady I had managed. Seamus reported that, in addition to the punctured lung, the abdominal surgery had revealed some perforated sections of bowel but nothing more. These had been repaired and she was stable and in the ward. We were about to move on when Seamus shifted in his chair and said, 'I'd like to make a general comment or two.' Everyone squirmed. Despite being a junior registrar, Seamus was competent and well respected. He had a gritty charm and a gruff demeanour that, combined with his charming accent, made him irresistible to most of the women in our group. He, in turn, was usually generous with his time and forgiving of mistakes. Unlike many of his fellow registrars, who preferred the thrill of theatre, he spent a lot of time with the interns in The Pit. Yet, for some reason, since the day I arrived, I had rubbed Seamus up the wrong way. Now it looked like he was displeased. And when he was displeased, people listened.

He cleared his voice. 'Note-taking is a key component of what we do here. They are medico-legal documents and should be treated as such. So when I see notes on a trauma patient with only *one* recorded blood pressure and only *two* saturation measurements, it really is unacceptable.' He didn't look at me, but I knew it was my notes he was referring to. Everyone knew. I wished I could have told him about the lack of room space, about the broken equipment, about the million things that made the work so tough. But these excuses would not have impressed anyone because we all faced them on a daily basis. So I elected to remain silent.

'All the good work in the world is for nothing if it's not properly documented. Good and accurate notes benefit our patients, our colleagues, and our ... ah ... legal friends. Often, they're the only evidence we did anything at all.'

I could feel my cheeks going red and the sweat returning. Everyone wanted Seamus's approval (myself included), and here he was giving me a very public dressing-down. I could feel his eyes boring into my bowed head. 'Resuscitation notes are crucial and should reflect multiple values and measurements. We're not medical students. I trust you all get the message.'

The drive home was surprisingly easy because I was powered by a mixture of shame and indignation. Shame that my best efforts had been used to teach others what *not* to do, by someone we all respected. Indignation because I felt I had been hard done by. Yes, the notes weren't perfect but the patient was alive and recovering. Wasn't that what mattered? I also couldn't shake the feeling that it wasn't that incident *per se* that had irritated Seamus but rather that it had been the spark that had ignited resentments that went way back. Seamus had been exasperated by my sparse note-taking; my over-reliance on my own clinical judgement rather than hard, objective measurements; my determination to spend more time with patients and less time with their files. I wasn't like him and his harsh words solidified in my gut that surgery and trauma weren't for me. But I also wished he had spoken to me privately rather than the public dressing-down. I vowed, in future,to raise my concerns with junior colleagues privately.

When I woke up later that day, I was completely disorientated. It was dark outside but all the lights in the house were on. As I groggily found my bearings, I realised that it was the evening, not morning. I sat up and tried to shake the heaviness from my eyes. Waking up from a long sleep and still feeling drained was something I was slowly adjusting to. My body had been running on pure adrenaline for twenty-four hours and was now having to manage with its sudden absence. In addition, my pineal gland was desperately trying to repair my damaged circadian clock, while the physical toll remained in my weary limbs. In short, I was a wreck. I was too jazzed to stay in bed, but the thought of getting up triggered an exhaustion I felt all the way to my bone marrow. Eventually, my full bladder forced me to get up and go to the bathroom. On the way back, I checked my phone. Two new messages: one from Mandy, the other from Lucy.

Hey sweets. Let's meet up soon? You looked a bit rough the other day! Maybe some TLC is needed ... xoxo

Mandy had been dancing around me for weeks, managing to avoid any firm plans for a date, but sending cute texts whenever I was about to give up. I gave it some thought and then responded.

A bit broken, tbh. Call super rough. Wanna go out and grab a drink?

The second text was from Lucy. We had been hanging out and

intermittently hooking up when we were both free. Despite my assertions that I was not looking for anything serious, she continued to ask me over. I tried not to overthink this arrangement. She knew the rules of a 'friends-with-benefits' relationship, I told myself, and then immediately winced when I thought about the preceding weekend. In bed, after sex, she had rolled over and said, 'Al ... what *is* this? We've been seeing each other for a few weeks now, but I have no idea what's going on.'

I should have seen this coming, and yet, astonishingly, I hadn't. The culture shock of work had been so overwhelming that I had barely had time to think at all. I suddenly felt panicked.

'Why do we need to label everything?' I had responded lamely. The words were as disingenuous and insincere coming out of my mouth as they were in my head, but it was too late. I tried to recover. 'I know it's cliché, but seriously, can't we just not worry too much about this stuff?' I could see she had been unimpressed, but didn't want to pursue the topic, so she mercifully let it go. Since that moment, however, I knew that she was only putting up with our casual relationship in the hope that I would change my mind and that it would one day bloom into something more. Unfortunately, while I enjoyed the sex, I had no desire to escalate anything. My thoughts, mostly, were on Mandy.

Hey Mr, Lucy's text read. *You must be shattered! No pressure, but if you wanna come and chill, we can watch Batman Begins and eat an entire tub of ice cream. And then, if you want, we could find a way to burn off those calories ...*

This was our familiar pattern, and in my state, the idea of cuddles, junk food and sex seemed mightily appealing. But just at that moment, Mandy texted back. This was unusual; she usually kept me waiting much longer for responses.

I love the idea of hanging out! Let's make it dinner? After the lunch thing last week, I feel like we need some time! Your choice?

The 'lunch thing' she was referring to was a braai at Angela's place. It was supposed to be a relaxed gathering of the interns, but Mandy had arrived nearly three hours late, and had then flirted brazenly with one of the orthopaedic registrars, before dashing off without saying a word to me.

Heart thudding, I named a nearby Italian place and we agreed to meet in just over an hour. I flung myself into a scalding shower and tried to wash the dark bags from under my eyes. I threw on an outfit I thought made me look cute and I dashed out the door. It would be tight, but if traffic was kind I should be able to make it, I thought.

I arrived and got us a table for two near the window. Despite the rush, everything was perfect. The table was private, the ambience was romantic, the music not too loud. I ordered a Sprite and waited.

Fifteen minutes after our meeting time, I began to worry. I checked my phone. Nothing.

At thirty minutes, I sent a message:

Everything ok? Do I need to send a rescue party?

At forty-five minutes:

Seriously, I'm worried. You ok?

By now, I was receiving pitying looks from the waiter. 'Are you still expecting anyone? The kitchen closes in an hour ...'

I mustered a smile and murmured, 'Traffic, ya know? It can be bad in Jozi.' I don't think either of us bought it.

Eventually, an hour later, my phone buzzed. I saw the text was from her and dreaded opening it.

Hey sweets. I'm SOOOOOOOOOOO sorry. I work for the SPCA in my spare time, and we had an emergency regarding a dog that was being abused. Don't think I'll be able to make it tonight ...

I turned the phone over in disgust before reading the rest.

She had stood me up. When I stopped at the garage shop on the way home, the freezer had malfunctioned from electricity blackouts that had suddenly hit the country, and all the ice cream had melted.

Working in trauma meant one twenty-four-hour shift in The Pit, followed by three days in the ward. The ward days were long: 'Pre-rounds' with the registrars began at 7am, followed by the 'Consultant' rounds at 11am. In theory, there was supposed to be time between the two to allow us to do the work identified on the 'Pre-round', but often the ward was so full that one round bled into the other.

If working in The Pit was the drama-filled party night, working the ward was the hangover. Inserting a drain to save someone's life is dramatic, removing it once it has served its purpose far less so. There were always so many people filling the beds that forming any sort of bond was impossible. The minute their lives were no longer in actual danger, they were discharged.

Except for the Vegetable Patch.

The Vegetable Patch was the (unkind) name given (no one knows by who) to the corner of the ward filled with patients with severe head injuries. These were people who had enough brain function that they did not require machines to keep them alive, but not enough that they were able to take care of themselves. Given how challenging and time-consuming it was to look after someone in this state, many had been abandoned by their families. Some had never been claimed at all. On my first day working in that area, I noticed that many were called either 'Sipho Vilakazi' or 'Thandi Vilakazi'. The registrar explained that this was the equivalent of 'John or Jane Doe'; someone whose name we had never found out. Many died still bearing their Baragwanath-anointed name.

Caring for patients in the Vegetable Patch quickly became something I enjoyed. For one, it was quiet. Or as quiet as a ward at

Baragwanath was ever going to be. There were only a few beeping monitors, minimal noisy foot traffic and little conversation. Even the pastors and preachers, who routinely strode between the beds promising salvation, were nowhere to be found. Almost like they had realised their words were wasted here. The only thing I hated about this area was its name. Reducing these patients to vegetables felt disrespectful.

'What would you call it instead?' one of the surgical registrars said. 'And who cares anyway? It's not like we're hurting their feelings or anything.'

'How about something nice?' I said.

'What about "Clifton Beach"?' Angela suggested.

'I dunno ... it still feels like we're teasing them, and I don't want to do that,' I responded. 'Maybe ... Magnum Lane?'

'What a weird name. Why that one?' The registrar was confused.

'I dunno. Magnums are my favourite ice cream. I think it's cool.' Everyone shrugged and moved on. From then on the area became known as Magnum Lane.

Every day the ward round would typically zoom through Magnum Lane because, frankly, there was nothing exciting or trauma-based to do. Every now and then one of the patients in the Lane would spike a fever, or need some oxygen, or choke on the secretions in the tubes in their necks, but for the most part, they simply lay there, unmoving. When they died, it was sometimes many hours before anyone even noticed.

When I was post-post-call (the day after being post-call, often worse than being post-call because you're still tired but expected to function fully), with a brain still buzzing from a long shift, I would head over to Magnum Lane to examine my patients. I took my time and tried my best to speak to them as if they were fully awake and conscious. I apologised to Sipho 4 if I had to poke him more than once to take blood. I asked Thandi 3 if she wanted to be moved into a ray of late afternoon sunshine that speared through the motes of hospital dust and settled next to her bed. And soon I began to realise that the unkind name originally given to this portion of the ward was, ironically, accurate. Vegetable patches are *alive*. They teem with life. From the bacteria and fungi and worms that populate the soil, to the birds and rodents, there is so much that goes on both above and beneath the ground. And so it was with the area formerly known as the Baragwanath Vegetable Patch.

Sipho 1 was definitely a morning person and became grumpy if I tried any procedures late in the afternoon. Thandi 3 grew lonely when her neighbour, Thandi 2, went for her daily physio sessions. Sipho 4 hated his catheter and was only mollified by a thigh rub. Thandi 1 loved the highveld thunderstorms and became noticeably more animated and happier the louder the pounding rain fell on the corrugated roof. These feelings were conveyed through subtle movements such as a squeeze of the hand, a jerk of the foot. They could be easily missed if you weren't looking out for them. I remember once asking one of the nurses if she also noticed and receiving a bemused laugh in return.

'Doctor, these patients can't think. There's too much brain damage. The neurologists say so. They just lie there. All this stuff is in your imagination. It's nice to believe they're responding to you, but I've been here for many years and, trust me, nothing changes.'

A few days after being stood up, I was woken by my alarm clock at 6am feeling completely flat. Every limb felt weighed down and when I eventually rose from bed and went into the bathroom, the reflection staring back at me in the mirror was not pretty. My thick, curly hair – difficult to control at the best of times and usually kept

PART 1: THE PRESENTATION

short to avoid maintenance – was flailing all over my scalp. My eyes were bloodshot and had dark rings under them. My skin, usually fairly clear, was reverting to my adolescent days and had broken out in an angry conflagration of pimples and blackheads. A scalding shower failed to help me feel any better and when I emerged, I discovered that all my sets of scrubs were in the laundry basket.

Dr Petkov had made it clear on day one in trauma that we all had to wear the same navy-blue scrubs every day, so I was forced to ransack my dirty clothes, trying to find the set that was the least offensively smelling and rumpled.

All my shoes were spattered with blood and couldn't be worn in that state, which meant I had no choice but to throw on my ugly pair of Crocs. I had vowed I would only ever wear them on overnight shifts, when no one was around to see them, but today I was simply out of options.

So it had to be that in this abject state, I bumped into Mandy.

As always, she was looking radiant. Her perfect hairstyle looked like she had come straight from the hairdresser. Her make-up and outfit were flawless. Crooked grin – which she flashed the moment she saw me – as knee-buckling as ever. I tried to look for an exit to scurry down as she approached me in the corridor, but there was nowhere to go. I exhaled and then realised with horror I had forgotten to brush my teeth.

'Hey sweets! How're you? You've been so quiet recently.'

'Yeah, um, you know ... being stood up will kind of do that to you, I think ...' I tried to sound angry, but without opening my mouth too wide. I came off more like a wounded puppy. I looked down and tried to straighten my rumpled shirt.

'Aw ... are you mad at me? Seriously, I'm so sorry. But that poor dog needed help and there was *literally* no one else. What was I supposed to do?'

Suddenly, I found I was doubting myself. Had this all been a terrible misunderstanding? Was I making this situation all about me and my hurt when, really, an abused animal needed help? And more importantly, if she hadn't really stood me up then surely she would be keeping her distance. Was her talking to me now evidence that there was still interest there?

'Look, let me make it up to, okay? Maybe we can hang out after work? I've heard you make an *amazing* lasagne.'

'Who told you that?'

'Word gets around.' She winked and I thought my bones would collapse.

'I'll think about it,' I tried to scowl.

'Unless you're done with me and want to see other people?' There was an edge to her question; a desire to probe. We hadn't even had a proper date yet so it had never occurred to me that I owed her exclusivity. Nevertheless, thoughts of Lucy flashed through my mind, and I felt inexplicably exposed. Disorientated, I could only mumble, 'No, of course not. You're such a force of nature it's hard to think about – let alone date – anyone else.' I regretted the lie immediately; it seemed so unnecessary. Before I could express that my existing love life was really none of her business, she grinned and said, 'Oh, sweets. You have such a way with words. It makes me crazy-fuzzy ...' She pecked my cheek and skipped off into the ward.

'You're a fucking idiot, you know that?'

'I agree. You're not thinking. As usual.'

Kobus and Angela were not pulling any punches.

I was on the defensive. 'What was she supposed to do? Just ignore an abused puppy? You know how much she loves animals. She could never just stand by while one was in pain.' I wasn't sure where the urge to defend Mandy had come from, but I suddenly felt righteous.

'Please tell me you're not buying that bullshit story? A bloody *puppy*? In *Pretoria*? And there was no else who could go ...?' Kobus was disbelieving.

'She's playing you, I'm afraid.' Angela sounded as certain as one of her diagnoses.

'Then why was she so keen to try to make it up to me? Wouldn't she want to avoid me for a while?' I countered.

'Ja, that's pretty weird. Chicks are weird,' said Kobus. We all nodded sagely.

At that moment, my phone pinged. Hoping it was Mandy firming up the evening plans, I glanced at it. It was a message from Lucy.

Hey Mr. What's going on? You're being all weird and distant. Every time I think we're going somewhere, you pull away. So I'm going to try one more time. Wanna hang at mine tonight?

It was 3pm, and I still hadn't heard from Mandy. A sudden flash of anger surged through me. Why risk another evening staring at my phone when I was guaranteed company with Lucy?

Sure, can I bring anything?

Just your appetite, followed by a winking emoji.

The Pit, which had been sedate that morning, was suddenly filled with the bustle of footsteps and the squeak of stretcher wheels. The nurses called us to the resus bay; four people had been caught in a shack fire. These were a sadly common occurrence during the highveld winters, when the combination of fires and heaters for warmth, intense dryness and densely packed, highly flammable structures, made rapid and devastating fires a constant and terrifying prospect.

To this day, I have nightmares about the burns we used to see. Being seriously burned is one of my deepest fears.

It was immediately apparent that we were fighting a losing battle. All four patients had more than ninety per cent burns covering their bodies. Their chance of survival was essentially zero. Human beings need skin not only to stop outside pathogens entering our bodies, but to maintain warmth, and to stop all our fluids leaking out. When that much of it has burned away, there is little that can be done, especially with our limited resources.

Seamus arrived, having been summoned from the ward to assist. When he walked in and saw what had arrived, it was as if he were a balloon suddenly deflated.

I was trying to insert an IV line through the ruined skin of one of the patients, always surprised by how cool deep burns feel to the touch – as if the warmth of human flesh has been charred away, leaving something alien and cold. I eventually found some unburned flesh around the patient's clavicle and managed to insert a long central line.

'They all need to be intubated,' Seamus said. There was charring around the patients' noses and lips, indicating that the flames had damaged their airways, which would soon swell shut if we didn't get something inside to help them breathe.

We set up the equipment and slipped the endotracheal tubes into their throats, which were already showing signs of closing. We didn't have enough ventilators available in the ICU, so in cases like this we simply connected the tubes to oxygen in the wall.

'Give them morphine!' he commanded.

'How much?' I asked. He stopped and looked at me. 'As much as they bloody well need.'

The burn team arrived shortly afterwards and confirmed what we all suspected. Their chance of survival was zero and there was no point in them being admitted to the burn unit as there was nothing they could do to change this. The best option was to send

PART 1: THE PRESENTATION

them to the trauma ward with fluids and morphine and wait for the inevitable. In the meantime, the extended family had arrived. Seamus and I accompanied them to the ward along with the patients. They were in shock. A young woman, a niece of one of the patients, knelt by the bed.

'They were just trying to stay warm. You know how cold it is. Their heater was old and the blanket got too close. And now ...' Tears spilled down her face.

'How long do they have?' she asked.

I told her I wasn't sure, but that it could take a while. Hours, days perhaps. This brought on a fresh wave of sobs. A middle-aged man, the son, asked me sternly what we were doing for his father. I explained that the tube would stop his throat from swelling shut, that the fluids would keep him hydrated, and the morphine would dull the pain.

'So, what will happen?'

I shifted uncomfortably on my feet. 'Eventually, he'll lose too much fluid and his body will shut down. Or he'll get an infection because his skin can't keep the bugs out.'

'Is he suffering?'

'We're doing our best with the morphine, but it's a really severe burn. It's very difficult to remove all the pain completely.'

'Can't you give him more?'

'Well ... we're at the maximum dose already. It's not safe if we go beyond that.'

He frowned. 'I don't understand. You said he's going to die anyway ... so why are you worried about a bit too much pain medicine?'

Seamus came to the rescue. 'Because that's not how it works here. We can't do things that we know are harmful.'

There was an awkward pause. 'But ...', Seamus continued, '... if we were just turning it up to manage the pain ... and not for any other reason ...' He let the sentence dangle.

The son looked at his dad, shifting uncomfortably in the bed, then back at us.

'I think you should turn it up.'

By the time I left work, it was after 7pm. The dry air sucked all the moisture from my cracked lips. My constant exposure to the devastation wrought by fires on the patients we saw at the hospital made it feel as if there was something malignant lurking behind the brown grass and dusty roads of Soweto; an evil force waiting to strike at any time. It made me shiver. I pulled over at a petrol station to buy my usual energy drinks and slurped one down greedily as soon as I got back in my car. I put on the stereo and cranked up a song by The Parlotones, a mainstream South African rock band, while waiting for the caffeine jolt. I checked my phone for the first time since the burn patients had arrived that afternoon and saw that I had a Facebook notification. I was not particularly active on Facebook so this was a bit of a surprise. I clicked on the notification, hoping to see a poke from Mandy, or perhaps a cute private message. Anticipation turned to horror when I realised that Lucy had left a long and effusive message on my public Facebook wall: 'This handsome cutie is KICKING ASS as an intern and rocks my world! Can't wait 2 spend more time hanging out, discussing dorky medicine, and getting 2 know u better. Mwa!'

My heart jolted as both adrenaline and caffeine bounded through my veins. This was a disaster. I quickly scanned the message to see when it had been posted. 4:42pm. Two and a half hours ago. I could only hope Mandy hadn't seen it. Our conversation from earlier that day was fresh in my mind and once again I cursed my stupidity. Why hadn't I just been honest about seeing Lucy occasionally? Now I was trapped in a lie and I had to do something.

PART 1: THE PRESENTATION

I knew from the frequency of her Facebook updates that Mandy was a regular visitor on the site so it was only a matter of time before she saw the post. But I also knew that Lucy had posted for a reason: she was frustrated by my prevarications and wanted to plant a flag. To stake a claim. Anyone reading her post would think we were dating, and that was the point; she was making a move, and now it was my turn. If I 'liked' it, or better yet (from her point of view), responded positively with a public message, I would be affirming her claim.

What if I didn't do anything? Pretended it didn't exist? I was only intermittently on Facebook anyway so there was plausible deniability. But on reflection, I realised that that wouldn't work either because sooner rather than later Mandy would see it. And my lie to her would be exposed.

Shit.

By the time I got home, I had formulated a plan. Once in my room I opened the site, clicked the thumbs-up icon to show I had 'liked' the post, and then, as surreptitiously as possible, I designated her post as 'private', hiding it from public view. When it was done, I exhaled slowly. Now I just had to hope that Lucy wouldn't notice.

She noticed immediately. Less than ten minutes after I hid the post, she called me and in a stern tone said that we had 'reached our sell-by date'. Although she was doing her best to maintain her composure, I could hear the tears behind the anger. She hung up before they could burst through.

I had a sick feeling in my stomach. How had I managed to turn 'friends with benefits' into more pain? I decided I needed distracting. I texted Mandy.

Any chance you're up for lasagne at mine tomorrow?

Thirty seconds later she responded.

Could think of nothing I'd like more, sweets.

I was not a good cook. I lacked the natural ability that so many people have when it comes to handling food in the kitchen, but there were a few dishes I could make competently and one of them was a lovely, cheesy lasagne. I had memorised the recipe the year before and had practised making it enough that I knew it was a winner. Friends who routinely derided my lack of culinary finesse were forced to concede that when it came to this dish, I knew what I was doing.

The bad news was that it took a lot of effort. The key was the sauce; I used two different types of tomato and onions, beef and garlic. While getting the pasta sheets ready, I usually prepared three types of cheese for the sauce: ricotta, Parmesan and mozzarella. Because we were out of Parmesan at home, I dashed to the shops to get some. When I got back home, I painstakingly layered the sauce and pasta sheets, making sure to get the balance between the sauce and the cheese just right. When everything was ready, it went in the oven to cook through.

I rushed up to my room and shaved for the first time in days. I hadn't had time to visit a barber in weeks and the back of my neck was hairy. I had always been self-conscious about this so I shaved it, trying my best to do it blindly. When I was ready, I scrubbed myself down, threw on my best shirt, splashed on some cologne and ran downstairs just as the oven alarm went off.

The lasagne looked delicious. The cheese had melted with just the right amount of crunch along the edges. The sauce had cooked through and the pasta had a pleasing al dente firmness to it.

I set the table and got a DVD ready in case Mandy wanted to relax after dinner. I chose *Horton Hears a Who* because she had once mentioned she was a huge Dr Seuss fan.

At 8pm, I was ready. My legs were jiggling in anticipation but I

PART 1: THE PRESENTATION

knew Mandy would be impressed. Hell, I was impressed. I had also barely thought of Lucy all day, which was a relief because the guilt still knotted my stomach. Mandy hadn't texted, but she knew my address and I was confident she would arrive soon.

She never arrived.

Initially, I was in denial. Had she been in an accident? Maybe hijacked? My mind was spinning. Jozi could be a dangerous city.

In the end, it was more banal than that. Something better came up for her. She never admitted it, of course, but there are only so many dogs in Pretoria that need rescuing on a weekend night. I tried calling but she didn't answer, and the voice note she sent a few hours later had a slightly drunken lilt to it.

I wasn't sure whether to be angry at her or mad at myself. The signs had been there; I had been warned. Nevertheless, it was still desperately deflating. With Lucy having dropped me, I had pinned my hopes on Mandy. That had clearly been foolish, and I felt like a fool. I knew I would never hear the end of it at work and I was dreading facing down my colleagues on Monday.

Sometimes you just need your mum. This was one of those times.

'How was your week?' she asked as we sat eating my beautiful lasagne. It steamed as I shovelled it into my mouth. Some sauce spilt on my fresh shirt, but I didn't care. I recounted everything that had happened. The exhaustion. The stress. The pressure. The banal and the serious. Pain and death juxtaposed with quotidian girl troubles. End-of-life decisions interspersed with sneaky Facebook shenanigans. Bottomless grief and foiled romances. You couldn't make this stuff up.

When I had finished my mum shook her head. 'Being a junior doctor in this country is crazy ...'

Chapter 7
ACTIVE LABOUR

Prayer time in the labour wards at Baragwanath was serious business. Every woman, regardless of her stage of delivery, was shepherded from her location to the row of chairs in front of the sisters' desk. There, the morning hymns would be sung, prayers to the Almighty offered, and the daily nursing updates 'delivered' (everyone enjoyed this little pun). While the singing and praying had been peaceful and moving in the medical and surgical wards, the effect in the labour wards was somewhat different. The beautiful hymns were frequently interrupted with groans, sighs and yelps as women dealt with the pain of imminent delivery. 'Amazing Grace' feels and sounds very different when women are yelling, 'Yhooooooo!' or 'Haw' weh ma' or 'Baby's coming!' during the chorus. The nurses forged on, undeterred, and I only ever saw proceedings halted on one occasion. That was when the baby's head emerged from under the mother's gown during the second verse. She was quickly shuffled away, and after a brief pause the hymn continued.

For reasons that aren't clear, more deliveries happen at Baragwanath in September than any other month, or at least that was the case when I was working there. Some speculate that many poorer South Africans, working in the big cities, return home over the Christmas holidays, reuniting them with partners they may not have seen for months. Others believe that the general festivities and merriment of the New Year naturally lead to more romantic liaisons. But even by September standards, this year was particularly busy. Eli, one of the new interns, who was big into astrology, claimed it had something to do with Aquarius being in retrograde during the previous December, which heralded a fertile phase. Phelo muttered that we were a cursed year, doomed to have the worst of everything. Regardless, by the time we entered our obstetrics and gynaecology block (the final one of the year), any thoughts of a reprieve from the hectic schedules of medicine and surgery were quickly banished.

Obstetrics at Baragwanath has its own building, sequestered, much like pregnant women of old, in a corner of the hospital far away from public view. Obs took up three of the four months of the rotation (the final one was spent in gynaecology), and interns were divided into four teams, with each team on call every fourth night. The other days were spent recovering from call duty, managing women admitted with obstetric complications (pre-eclampsia, high blood pressure, gestational diabetes, etc.) or running the antenatal clinic. But call was the day around which the other days orbited. It meant arriving at 8am in the morning, seeing the patients in the ward and then trying to snatch some rest in the afternoon before the night shift started at 5pm. Some brave souls would try to sneak home; most of us just tried to find a quiet room with a desk in it so we could lay our heads down.

Being on obstetric call meant treating women who were in labour or who had just delivered. The labour ward was in an imposing brick building divided into four main sections: latent labour, active labour, post-delivery and theatre. Interns spent most of their time in the latent labour area and assisting in theatre with caesarean sections. The registrars spent their time in the active labour area, along with the midwives, or in theatre doing the bulk of the cutting.

Latent labour is that period when a woman is experiencing contractions, but her cervix hasn't dilated beyond four centimetres. Women can be in latent labour for a long time, and we had to manage them when they arrived. This meant clerking them in, assessing the pregnancy with manual palpation of the abdomen and ultrasound scans, and performing vaginal examinations to assess the extent of the cervical dilation. If women were less than four centimetres dilated, they were sent to sit on a hard bench, and their names were entered into a big, tatty book that sat on a lectern at the room's entrance. They were reassessed in four hours and if they still weren't in the active phase, reassessed four hours again after that. If, after eight hours, they *still* weren't in active labour, they would be told to go home and return when the contractions became more severe. During busy periods there were often thirty or more women sitting cheek to cheek on the 'awaiting-to-be-reassessed' bench.

Once a woman progressed beyond four centimetres, she was considered to be in 'active labour' and was whisked away to the delivery area, where we wouldn't see her again unless there was a complication.

On my first call I asked one of the nurses why there weren't any beds, or at the very least, comfortable couches for the women in latent labour to rest on. She said that Bara didn't have enough beds for the women in *active* labour let alone those in latent. As for comfortable couches, they had tried that, but after the umpteenth woman's water broke all over the fabric, and after the umpteenth baby was delivered on them, they had been abandoned for hygienic purposes. All that remained were the long, lonely wooden benches,

PART 1: THE PRESENTATION

lined up side by side. Favoured because lacquered wood doesn't absorb bodily fluids.

In September of that year, Baragwanath was averaging over ninety deliveries every day. To keep up with demand, there were two theatres running 24/7 performing caesarean sections. This meant there was little to no registrar support or supervision in the antenatal areas.

I had been placed in a team with Jonathan (a Wits graduate), Phelo, Anwar and Lucy. Lucy still wasn't talking to me after the Facebook debacle, and when she was forced to interact for professional reasons, she'd stare over my shoulder while she relayed the pertinent information before hurrying off. I had never worked with Jonathan before but he immediately struck me as an unusual guy. My initial instinct was that beneath the conservative Afrikaner exterior, he was very obviously gay. Yet he kept mentioning how he was looking for a girlfriend. When I brought this up with Angela (who had studied with him at med school), she said that he *had* come out the closet in third year and then promptly jumped back in in fifth year. He had also been, at various stages, a Christian, an atheist and an orthodox Jew.

We were a diverse group of interns with every race, gender and religion represented. This made accommodating religious holidays very complicated. During this block, we celebrated Ramadaan, Diwali, Christmas, Boxing Day, Yom Kippur and various other holidays. Everyone wanted time off to enjoy their holy days, so hospital management said that all staff who were religious could take two days. When the non-religious interns asked about our provision, we were initially told that we couldn't take religious time off if we weren't religious. It was around that time that many of us 'rediscovered' our religious roots, or created humanistic holidays that we claimed as our own.

Jonathan said he was 'pan-religious' and hadn't decided which path he wanted to follow, but he wanted more than his allotted two days. In addition, he had very mixed feelings about working on weekends, he said. Depending on which religion he was 'feeling' in any given week, he might want Saturdays or Sundays (or both!) off.

Hospital management quickly stepped in and stressed that on-call work was essential and lifesaving and that he could not opt out. He grudgingly accepted this, but then said he could not do 'non-essential' ward work on weekends. Had Jonathan been excused it would have meant that the rest of us would have had to work every single weekend in the block. This was clearly unacceptable and unfair, so we objected. When Jonathan was told he had to work on weekends, he then said he was forbidden from driving on the Sabbath, which was how I found myself picking him up every Saturday morning to get to work. Not only did I have to chauffeur him, but I also had to open the car door for him as manipulating it turned on the inside light, which his understanding of his religion forbade him from doing.

The feeling among the interns quickly turned from one of wanting to assist a colleague observe and discover his sincerely held religious beliefs, to suspicion that he was wearing whichever religious 'hat' was most helpful at any given time to allow him to get out of work he clearly despised. Jonathan vehemently denied this insinuation but would claim every religious day – no matter how minor – as a reason not to come to work. His frequent absences put strain on the team and by the second month we were all even more exhausted. Jonathan himself appeared unhappy, and often missed days due to unspecified and vague medical ailments, which stretched our exhausted group further.

Our antipathy towards Jonathan was exacerbated by the fact

PART 1: THE PRESENTATION

that everyone was on edge and sleep deprived. Days smudged into days, patients smudged into patients and everything become dull and boring. The act of bringing life into the world – so wondrous when I had been a student – became monotonous and nondescript. Perhaps this was because we were hardly present for the deliveries themselves as patients disappeared the moment they progressed beyond the magic four-centimetre mark. Perhaps it was a long year catching up with us. Perhaps we were all just getting sick of spending every waking minute (and many sleeping ones, too) with each other. Perhaps we were all over Jonathan's nonsense. Regardless, the block felt like a drag.

The 'sleeping room' in obstetrics was a normal, standard-sized room with three cardboard partitions and beds with mattresses that smelled exactly as you'd expect a mattress that hundreds of other sweaty humans had slept on to smell. The 'walls' were so flimsy that every movement made in the room was audible to everyone else. Jonathan was a big guy and a loud snorer, and the small room amplified the terrific vibrations that emerged from his mouth while he was sleeping. It got so bad that one night, during a precious two-hour window of rest, I gave in and got up, bumping into a bleary-eyed Phelo, who had clearly also decided that sleep wasn't happening for him either.

'I'm not a violent person,' he said, 'but if my pillow weren't so damn flimsy, I'd suffocate him with it.' I nodded. I shared the sentiment.

During one of my shifts, I clerked in a woman who was having her eighth baby. I had assessed her and everything seemed to be on track. She was only three centimetres dilated and her contractions were relatively mild. I put her on the bench and marked her for

ACTIVE LABOUR

reassessment in four hours. She began groaning as soon as she sat down, but this wasn't unusual as the bench was uncomfortable and at any given time, sighs and moans could be heard coming from all directions.

Sister Albertina, a hardened warrior of the obstetric wards, who bore the battle scars and appeared years older than she really was, looked at the patient curiously and then came up to me.

'Dokotela, she looks familiar. What's going on?'

'Oh, nothing much. Latent labour. This is pregnancy number eight. I know these can progress quickly so we'll keep a close eye.'

Sister Albertina's eyes suddenly filled with panic. 'Number eight! Hawu! Get the wheelchair RIGHT NOW! We need to get her to delivery. Porter!'

As if by magic, a porter appeared, ready to take her.

'Hang on!' I yelped. 'She needs an IV or they won't accept her!'

'Then do it on the way, Dokotela! She's going to deliver!'

I couldn't believe my ears. Fifteen minutes ago she was still in latent labour. This was an overreaction, surely?

I decided to check the woman again just before we loaded her onto the wheelchair. It took me a minute to compute what my hand was feeling. The baby's head. The whole head. Somehow, she had fully dilated in ten minutes and the baby's arrival was imminent.

'Oh shit! Get her going!' I gesticulated to the porter. Time was of the essence because if she delivered in the antenatal area, we would face stern questioning and mountains of paperwork. Sister Albertina knew this and was witnessing her 9pm nap disappearing before her eyes in a mountain of documentation. Just the week before, a woman had delivered into the toilet because she had been waiting so long. Although the baby was fine, management was displeased and had informed us there was no excuse for that to happen again.

We got our patient to the labour ward just in time. She was

transferred to her bed, and with a grunt, a baby suddenly appeared and began howling angrily. Mostly, we were relieved she hadn't delivered on the wheelchair. I was about to head out when the nurse called me back. Something was wrong. The woman (whose name I had never caught) was moaning softly. But there was a different timbre to this sound, a plaintiveness missing from the pain of childbirth.

I looked down and saw that blood was pooling around the bed. She was bleeding profusely, probably because her uterus, after the eighth delivery, wasn't contracting sufficiently. This was a major post-partum haemorrhage and we were in trouble.

I asked the midwife if she had delivered the placenta because the main reason the uterus fails to contract is the placenta remaining behind, but she showed it to me, intact, in all its slimy glory. Meanwhile, the baby and its angry cries had been whisked away. I felt the mother's abdomen but could not palpate the uterus. This was unexpected.

As if by magic, a green tray appeared next to me. When Sister Albertina opened it, I saw dozens of gleaming instruments: speculums, scissors, forceps, suturing needles. This was the 'post-partum pack', something I hoped I'd never have to see. I told the midwife to call the registrar immediately but was informed she was busy in theatre. There was no one to help. I used a speculum to try to see what was going on. I was confronted with pools and pools of blood. When I tried to use gauze to stem the flow, I only had a clear vision of the vaginal canal for less than a second before the blood reaccumulated. But that one second was enough. The problem wasn't the uterus; it was her cervix. It was badly torn and bleeding profusely. I grabbed some sutures and gauze and muttered again, 'Where's the reg?'

At that moment I heard a loud crash as the door to the ward

burst open. A stretcher was being pushed in. I glanced round and saw a woman positioned on all fours, with Phelo in a similar pose behind her, his entire fist and wrist disappearing inside her vagina. I knew that meant only one thing: cord prolapse. The umbilical cord had emerged before the baby, which would cut off its blood supply. This was immediately life-threatening. The solution in this case was an urgent caesarean section, and the only way to buy time was to push the cord back in and then lift the baby's head off the pelvic floor to relieve the pressure. The one thing keeping the blood flowing to the baby was Phelo's fist, which was why he couldn't move. This wasn't the first time I had seen a case like this, and I knew it would take priority over my emergency. With a sinking feeling, I knew the reg wasn't coming to help. She would be in theatre fixing the cord prolapse for at least another thirty minutes.

I returned to the task at hand. Blood was pooling around my feet and Sister Albertina was hanging up a unit of O negative blood. She hardly ever looked nervous, but she had gone pale and quiet. The bottom line was that I had to stop the bleeding. I knew what had to be done, I just couldn't see what I was doing.

Sometimes in medicine doing something not very well is better than doing nothing. I identified a rough area of the cervix and began suturing. The needle disappeared into the blood and I wasn't sure whether I was even stitching anything, but I was in the right area and I had no choice but to keep trying. In my tired, but adrenaline-fuelled state, I knew I had to be careful or I would prick myself. The thought popped into my brain that I didn't know the patient's HIV status. But I did know that, at that time, upwards of thirty per cent of the women delivering at Bara were HIV-positive.

My hands were soon slick with blood, but after four or five stitches, the bleeding began to let up. Mercifully, I could see. My ragged sutures were ugly, but they had contained the bleeding. I

PART 1: THE PRESENTATION

quickly finished as best I could, checked her vital signs, and sent her to the high-care area for monitoring. I then decided I needed a cigarette.

Over the course of the year, I had treasured the brief moments of respite that sneaking away for a quick smoke offered. For a few minutes, I could step outside the chaos, get my jolt of inhaled nicotine, and do some reflection. I knew how bad it was for my physical health, but in that crazy year I didn't care. I was young and strong; I could focus on quitting another time.

As I approached the outside corridor, I could almost taste the acrid fumes already. This was one I would enjoy.

As I lit up, away from the sights and smells of the ward, I saw a silhouette, which turned out to be Phelo. He didn't smoke so it was unusual to see him outside like this.

'Looked like you had a bit of drama. Cord prolapse?' I asked.

'Ja,' he responded. 'Got her to theatre and she's being cut right now. I'll check on her and the baby when it's all over. Just needed some fresh air.'

'Yup. Same. I had a bad post-partum haemorrhage. Blood everywhere. Sorted now.'

'Cool, man. Nice one. When I go check on my lady, I'll see if yours is okay. What's her name?'

I suddenly realised that in all the chaos, I hadn't checked her basic details. 'I don't know,' I replied. 'I'll check when I get back inside.'

'Isn't it *weird* that you don't know? You clerked her, performed invasive exams and then saved her life, and you don't know her name?'

I bristled. 'Look, man. It was hectic in there. Between the delivery and the haemorrhage, there wasn't a lot of time for introductions.'

'Sure. I mean, okay. I just think it's a bit sad.'

'What is?' I was fully on the defensive now.

'What this place has done to us,' he said softly.

'What do you mean? I think the training we've had has been brilliant. Where else in the world would you have two *interns* managing life-threatening complications like that? And we fucking kicked ass!'

'But at what cost?' Phelo asked quietly.

'Sorry?'

'At what cost?' he repeated.

'I don't understand. They're both probably going to be okay.'

'I meant at what cost to *us*?' He paused. 'Do you remember that very first night we were on call for Ward 30? I remember seeing you outside. You were a wreck. You could barely clerk a patient; your IV lines were a hot mess. I honestly wasn't sure you'd make it the first week. But here's the thing: you knew every one of your patients' names. It was weirdly impressive ... and they liked you for it! Now, sure, you're good at procedures, and your IVs are *much* better, but you don't know everyone's name any more.'

'Dude, that's not fair. We clerk like a hundred patients every night. Do you know all their names?'

'I know the name of the lady who just had a cord prolapse. Portia Mashaba. She's thirty-three and from Diepsloot, but that's not the point. This is not about *you*, it's about this place,' he gestured around him, 'and what it takes from us. I'm not sure it's worth it. Because you know what? I miss the guy from Ward 20 who knew everyone's name.'

'Well, if that guy who could barely site an IV had been here tonight, I would probably be filling out a death certificate right about now.' I flicked the cigarette butt away and stormed back inside.

PART 1: THE PRESENTATION

The rest of the night was an endless parade of pelvic exams. I found that assisting with caesarean sections in theatre was boring and uncomfortable – the hot white lights, the thick sterile gowns, the sore feet ... and so I generally volunteered to continue in the labour ward or manage issues in the post-partum area.

When the sun came up, I dashed down to the ward to see the inpatients so that I could go home immediately after handover. I was dog-tired, but adrenaline coursed through my body; the rising sun had a way of energising me. It was a sign that home time was near. I absorbed its meagre warmth and got a second wind.

In the ward, I bumped into Mandy who was covering the weekend for her team and looked miserable. Light, which usually seemed to bend towards her, now seemed to arc away. She looked tired and haggard and there were dark rings patterned under her eyes. Although I personally hadn't felt like this in a long time, I knew immediately what was going on: Mandy was hungover.

Interns have never been saints. We all went out during the week, and functioning the next day on minimal sleep with a bit of a headache was common. But this, I knew, was different. This was the feeling of rotten egg yolk in a hard shell; a pressure that squeezed the back of your eyeballs; the taste of bile folding itself into your throat; a nausea that burrowed into your bones. Mandy had developed a reputation for skipping rounds. She usually got away with it because the male registrars were wrapped around her finger. One weekend in surgery, she had skipped ward call on a flimsy pretence, and not only had the registrar stood in for her, he had bought her flowers and a present the next day to show his solicitude. But the hard female registrars in obstetrics weren't buying it.

A civil truce had been declared between us. We joked and teased each other, and occasionally texted, but I had done my best to dampen down the intense spark I felt. By now, she was unpopular with the other female interns, who had grown increasingly irritated with her unreliability, and who felt she charmed her way out of facing any consequences for her erratic work ethic.

'You look like you could use some coffee,' I said.

'God, yes. Got any?'

'No. But I know where to find the best watered-down, instant stuff in the whole of Soweto. Don't say you aren't tempted.'

She smiled weakly. 'I accept.' Then she added, 'Got an aspirin?'

'No. But I have something better. I know a spot. A quiet spot.'

And so we found ourselves drinking bland coffee out of Styrofoam cups, standing in the makeshift marijuana patch, as the orange Gauteng sun crept up over the horizon. The leaves had withered and dried out after a harsh winter, but in the September spring there were some unmistakeable signs of life. The soil, previously dry and parched, now had a softness to it after welcome rains. Small, green buds were inching their way from the resurgent branches. It wasn't much but after a night under harsh fluorescent lights it felt like something.

'How do you know about spots like these?' Mandy asked. 'It's like some weird gift you have.'

'What do you mean?'

'Finding the nooks and crannies everyone else misses. That sunny patch in Magnum Lane, that warm closet in The Pit? It's like a gift.'

'Nah. Prof Waters just plants his weed here. He told me about it. No detective work required.'

'Well, no one else seems to know.' She glanced at one of the plants with its distinctive five-leaf shape. 'Ever been tempted?'

'I can't ...'

'Oh shit, yeah, that's right. I knew about the no drinking. But no other drugs either?'

PART 1: THE PRESENTATION

'No, nothing that alters my mind. Besides, weed was never my thing and I never tried the harder stuff.' I paused. 'Are you okay?'

'Me? Sure. Why do you ask?'

'We all have our "off days". It just seems to me that you've been having a lot of them recently.'

'Well, you know Manhattan ... can't leave until the 2am bangers have played.'

'But you were like this on Wednesday. Monday, too, if memory serves. Manhattan isn't open on Sundays.'

She suddenly sensed where I was going and tensed up. 'Are you keeping tabs on me? And so what if I did? God. Not everyone at this place likes to live here. Some of us can't *wait* to get out and have some fun. To forget. To have conversations that don't revolve around our patients, or our calls, or our dreadful sleep patterns. Or fucking TB. Some of us just want to have fun like normal people without having to answer a million questions about it every weekend.'

'I'm sorry, I didn't mean to interrogate you. I'm just concerned, that's all.'

But her hackles were raised. 'I just don't get this obsession with work. This place is so all-encompassing it's like we've forgotten that people go out and get shit-faced every now and then. That's normal. Know what's *not* normal?' She gestured vaguely around her.

'It just seems to be happening quite a lot, is all ...' I muttered, feeling increasingly foolish. 'Some of us are concerned.'

'Concerned? Or enjoying the gossip?'

'Concerned.'

'Don't worry about me, I'm fine. You're not my supervisor. Or my dad.' She walked away, but as she passed one of the healthier plants she stopped and gently rubbed one of its leaves.

'Sometimes I think you'd be a lot more fun if you smoked some of this.' Then she was gone.

'My car!' Anwar was distraught. 'It's gone!'

'What do you mean?'

'I mean, gone! Stolen! I left it here last night and it's not here any more.'

'Okay, don't panic. Maybe you parked it somewhere else and just got confused. I often don't remember exactly where I parked. I'm sure it's here somewhere.'

After ten minutes of searching, it became apparent that it was not, in fact, 'here somewhere'. Even more worrying was the shards of broken glass scattered around, indicating that a car window had likely been broken.

Anwar's car was his baby. A deep-blue BMW he had received from his dad, he spent a lot of time maintaining and caring for 'Jasmine', as he called her. Now Jasmine had been abducted.

He contacted his tracking service, who informed him that the alarm had been disabled and the tracker removed. They had no idea where the car was.

'Fuuuuuckkk,' was all he could muster.

'Look, don't panic, there are cameras all around the hospital and no one can leave without going through a security boom,' I said. 'Someone will have seen something.'

Security was about as helpful as one might expect. We were met with blank looks and non-committal shrugs. No one knew anything, and all the guards on overnight duty had gone home. The day team had nothing to add. Anwar was apoplectic.

'The car can't fly! It had to leave through one of the three exits! Someone from last night must've seen something! How does this happen?!'

'We'll ask around but we didn't hear of any unusual activity,' the head guard said.

On a normal day, Anwar would've probably walked away at this point, but the lack of sleep had removed his inhibitions.

'Let me get this straight: you guys are awesome at searching boots for a handful of essential supplies but you can't tell if an actual car has been *stolen*?'

Another shrug.

'What about CCTV footage? You guys have cameras, right?'

'We do but you need special hospital permission to access the material. The footage gets wiped every twenty-four hours, so you should get moving.'

As we trudged towards the monolithic administrative building, I felt like crying. Our beautiful, precious, post-call day was evaporating in front of our eyes and there was nothing we could do about it.

Chapter 8

BROTHERS IN ARMS

THE FINAL MONTHS OF INTERNSHIP FELT SURREAL. AFTER NEARLY TWO YEARS AT Bara it was time for most of us to move on. Between the clinic work at Chiawelo, psychiatry at Bara with a broken ankle (when you have to 'crutch' your way through the corridors you realise how vast it is), anaesthetics, more marches for better conditions in Pretoria and, of course, paediatrics, the second year had flown by. Now, having completed our 'apprenticeship', we were fully qualified doctors and able to practise independently. There was only one catch: community service.

Community service is an initiative that was introduced by the South African government in 1998. The idea was that doctors who had been heavily subsidised during their medical training should 'pay back' that support by working in a rural area for a year. This was intended to bolster medical services in parts of South Africa that had been neglected and where few physicians wanted to go.

Much like internship, applying for community service posts was a stressful and seemingly arbitrary process. You indicated your preferred hospitals on a form and were then assigned to one of them by a faceless bureaucrat, depending on supply and demand. For people who had established lives and homes in certain areas this could be tremendously disruptive. Some had partners they didn't want to leave behind; others a sick family member; others a trusted therapist whom they relied upon for their mental well-being. Most of us were in our mid-twenties by this stage, and simply uprooting everything for a year was disruptive and destabilising.

Nevertheless, there was a grudging acceptance that, from a public health perspective, the initiative had been a success. Many patients in far-flung corners of the country suddenly had access to a well-trained physician. And those willing to head into remote hospitals got experience and training they would not have received anywhere else.

I was completely undecided about whether I wanted to do adult medicine or paediatrics. I had recently completed my block of paediatrics and it had been every bit as fatiguing as adult medicine had been. But there was one key difference: when I arrived home after my days with adults, I frequently felt anger and frustration. Angry that I couldn't always provide them with the care they deserved because of resource limitations, and frustrated that I didn't have the time to work on the underlying issues that affected their health. Sadness that I was often so fatigued that I simply wanted them discharged to prevent my list from becoming even more overwhelming. Many of these issues were present during my paediatric block, but when I got home I felt neither angry nor sad. Rather, I was energised by the kids and their resilience and bravery, at the smiles they dished out with such generosity even when I'd hurt them while taking blood or inserting a urinary catheter. The ward rounds were very different to the ones I was used to in adult medicine. Gone were the intellectually stimulating discussions about esoteric conditions and deep dives into the minutiae of physiology (which I loved). These were replaced by issues some of my colleagues thought were banal: calculating the kids' intakes and outputs (often down to the millilitre of urine or the volume of stool), checking their vaccine status and assessing their developmental milestones. While perhaps not as 'intellectual', there was a charm and a joy to paeds that was missing in adult care. My head lay with the intricacies of the adult world, my heart with the joy of the paediatric one. I had to make a decision about where my future lay.

I figured I would use my 'comm serv' year to try to figure it out. I applied to every paediatric hospital in Gauteng and threw in some smaller, more peripheral areas as a back-up. I had one space left on the form and couldn't think of anywhere else I wanted to go, so I put down Baragwanath because I didn't feel like moving provinces again. But it was so far down the list that there was no way I would be coming back to Bara.

'You moron!' Phelo could barely contain his laughter. 'What's the thing we all learned in med school? You put Bara, you *get* Bara!'

I was staring numbly at my form. I had been placed in Chris Hani Baragwanath Hospital for another year. While many others would be saying their farewells, I would be staying behind. The sensation in my chest was an odd one; a mixture of confusion and a weird tinge of acceptance, as if a small part of me had always known that my dance with Baragwanath had not yet come to an end. I scanned down the list to see the rotations I had been assigned. The good news was that I would be able to do four months of paediatrics. The bad news was that to 'pay' for this I had to do some other rotations I was less enthusiastic about. I would be doing four months of general medicine and four months in the emergency room. It could've been worse.

PART 1: THE PRESENTATION

I would be joined by Anwar and Angela, who had purposefully stayed at Bara because they knew they would walk into a specialist training post if they could tough out another year in the adult medical wards. I was slightly jealous of the certainty they had about where their careers were going, but I also knew I had to be sure about the direction I wanted to take because I was so heavily conflicted.

On the last day of the year, the interns held a farewell party. It was strange saying goodbye to so many colleagues and friends I had worked with so closely during my two years at the hospital. We all felt as if we had survived a war together, and the looks were of frank relief rather than jubilation.

I couldn't help but notice some of the missing faces.

Samantha, who was so shell-shocked after her first intake in Ward 30 that halfway through the round the next day, she excused herself, jumped in her car, and never came back, leaving a fuming registrar in her wake.

Steve, who had fallen asleep at the wheel after a thirty-four-hour shift at the hospital, and had only just avoided gliding into one of Soweto's busiest intersections by the bumper of the car in front of him. He was so shaken that he had quit and gone into his father's cellphone business.

Portia, who had contracted multi-drug resistant TB from a patient and was rendered so unwell by the brutal regimen of medications and injections that she had taken indefinite sick leave.

Jemima, who had become so depressed that she had been forbidden by her concerned psychiatrist to return to work for three months.

The list went on.

The more I looked around, the more it became apparent that we were survivors rather than jubilant victors. People were glugging the alcohol in a desperate, almost angry manner. I sipped on my Coke, but was quietly envious about the oblivion some of my colleagues were entering. If people were having a great time, however, there was precious little evidence. Around me were smiles, but little laughter. Shared tales, but little nostalgia. Those of us who were remaining were met with glances of pity.

'Why did we never give it a proper go, sweets?'

Even after two years, and despite the fact that I was in a happy relationship by now, Mandy's voice always caught me off-guard. I turned round to face her, purposefully ignoring her hand gently resting on my shoulder. I tried to smile and appear relaxed.

'That's pretty forward. Isn't holding back and making people guess your next move more your style?'

There was a glint in her eyes and her eyebrows raised briefly in amusement. 'Touché.'

'I could ask you the same question,' I said.

She smiled. 'It wasn't a good time for me, but you were too angry to ever find out why. And you didn't take too long to move on anyway. I've seen your lady she's ... very pretty. But ...'

I knew it was a trap, that I should resist, but before I could help myself the words were out of my mouth. 'But what?'

'But ... aren't you a bit bored? Despite your goody-two-shoes persona you like to live on the edge. Deep down, you're drawn to the chaos. Like all addicts.'

'Maybe. But your brand of chaos made me sad. Plus, it's dangerous.' I noticed that her pupils were dilated even though the room was well lit. She was buzzing. I knew she was on something, but for some reason I didn't want to walk away.

'*Dangerous?*' She put her hand on her chest in mock horror. 'Oh my! Is that why you didn't try again?'

'I was busy. Not all of us had registrars wrapped around our fingers.'

PART 1: THE PRESENTATION

'Pfft. Nonsense.'

'Or maybe you didn't give me enough encouragement to keep it up? Or maybe I got tired of the rejection. Or maybe I realised you just liked the attention.' For the first time, I saw irritation skid across her lips, which were pursed. 'Or, maybe,' I continued, 'I realised I deserved better.'

She kept her eyes on me for a beat longer than was comfortable. 'You always were a bit different, sweets. You stand out. There's something about you I can't put my finger on. That's not a bad thing.'

'I'll bet you say that to all the boys.'

Again, the irritation flicked across her face. 'You make me sound like some kind of man-eater.'

'Well ... aren't you? I see how you use your looks to get what you want. I see how you flirt. You have plenty of disposable male interest. I don't think that I was any different.'

'You're talking shit.'

'Excuse me?'

'You heard me. You're talking shit. Do you have any idea what it's like being a woman in this place? Constantly being referred to as a "nurse" by patients, even when you correct them a million times? Having senior colleagues hit on you and ask for your number all the time? Having your medical decisions constantly undermined and questioned? It's fucking *exhausting*.'

'Shit, I'm sorry, I didn't mean to ...'

'Do you know why I stopped wearing scrubs? Because there are only men's sizes, and they have that enormous V-neck that hardly covers anything. The other day I was on a ward round in scrubs and one of the surgeons took out his phone, claiming he was messaging the anaesthetist, but then his bloody camera flashed.'

She saw the blank look on my face and sighed in exasperation.

'He was taking pictures of my fucking tits! Do you know how

humiliating that is? And I just had to take it while his colleagues sniggered. It's not just the interns, registrars get it too. It's endemic.'

My mind immediately wandered back to Chloe. That first medical block seemed so far away. After coming clean with me about Dr Simpson, Chloe had finished her rotation and had then taken an indefinite leave of absence. Everyone except me had been taken completely by surprise. No one knew the exact reason, but there were murmurings of 'personal issues' and 'boyfriend trouble'. I was ashamed to say that although we had parted on good terms, I hadn't kept in touch with Chloe. The hospital grind had churned so quickly that before I had time to breathe, I was in The Pit. I made a mental note to try to speak to Chloe at some point soon.

Mandy, meanwhile, had regained her composure. It was hard to tell whether she was more angry or sad. I also didn't know what to say, and if saying anything would just inflame the situation further. After a healthy sip of her wine, she continued. 'We all do what we can to get by in this place. Perhaps I wasn't always kind to you, and for that I'm sorry, but trying to be normal and have normal relationships when you have to put up with the kak this hospital throws at you day in and day out is so bloody hard.'

I swallowed. Hoping to lighten things up a bit, I asked what she was doing next.

'I got a scholarship to do some research at a hospital in America.'

'What? Oh my god! That's great! Right?'

'Ja. I need to get away. And this is a fabulous opportunity. I've always wanted to live abroad, you know?'

'See? Aren't you glad we didn't date? 'Cos now we'd have to break up.'

A tiny smile caressed her face. 'Doesn't mean there aren't regrets. But ja, I'm glad you're going to be here. It's right. I can feel it. You've changed, but there's still stuff you need to figure out.'

PART 1: THE PRESENTATION

The way she managed to intrigue me was both maddening and compelling. 'What do you mean?'

'I mean ... your brain isn't nearly as big as you think it is. You're at your sexiest not when you're being smart, but when you're sitting with those patients and you don't think anyone's watching. And the moment we all saw you in a paediatric ward with those laughing kids clamped around your legs we all knew where your future lay, even if you're still figuring it out.'

I gulped. 'I didn't think anyone saw that.'

Her laugh was as spontaneous as I had ever heard it and bounced off the walls. 'It's cute how blind you can be sometimes. When someone walks into a ward and three minutes later has children literally hanging off them, while the rest of the sick kids who haven't smiled in days are dissolving in laughter, you're onto something. And I could see it in your eyes. It was making you happy. Go be a great paediatrician.'

'I'm glad someone is so sure.'

Her phone buzzed. 'Gotta answer this. You take care.'

I never saw her again.

I did see Lucy, however. Things had remained frosty since our 'break-up'. She had started seeing a much younger guy, which made me weirdly jealous, but I knew I had no choice but to keep my mouth shut. She was heading to Cape Town for comm serv and I was secretly relieved I wouldn't have to duck and dive to avoid her in the corridors.

'Well, Mr Man, I wish I could say it's been a pleasure.'

'Yeah, I'm sorry. I was awful to you. You deserved better.'

'I did.' There was an awkward pause.

'I heard you were seeing someone. I'm happy for you,' I said.

'Thank you. He's a good guy.'

I thought that was the end of it and was making to move away, when she added, 'You've heard it before and you'll hear it again: you're the world's dumbest smart person. You think it's about your brain, but that just gets you into trouble. Follow that big heart of yours instead.' She gave me a peck on the cheek and was gone.

Saying goodbye to Phelo and Kobus was tough. We had spent so many nights together, gone through so many ward rounds, clinics and handovers, that bidding farewell felt strange. I had spent far more time with these guys in the past two years than I had with any friends or family. I had seen Kobus so tired he had crawled under a desk for somewhere flat to lie down. I had giggled deliriously and helplessly at Phelo stabbing himself in the eye with an invisible blade while a consultant ran through the causes of post-partum haemorrhage after we had barely sat down all night. A weird bond is formed when people work side by side at 3am, and I had never felt it stronger than at that moment. Not friendship exactly (I had never been to either of their houses and they had never come to mine. Social hangouts were limited to nights at Manhattan and group socials), but more like brothers in arms. Like an elastic band stretched to its limit, it felt both powerful and tenuous at the same time.

Phelo was heading off to do obstetrics in Limpopo. He wanted to ultimately go into obs and gynae and he had family living there. He had been accepted for a spot at one of the rural hospitals. Kobus was going back to Pretoria for a year of family medicine at one of the busy clinics there. His wife was pregnant again and he wanted to settle down and lay some roots.

We sipped our drinks and reminisced. About the chaos of Ward 30. About the horrors of The Pit. About falling asleep while delivering babies, about psychiatry, orthopaedics and family medicine. And how different we were as people two years later.

'I still feel like I know jack-shit,' Kobus laughed. 'I'm just better at *pretending* like I know what's going on. But I guess I know that I'm dumb about most stuff. Maybe that's what being a consultant is all about: knowing what you don't know.'

'I reckon I could get blood from a stone,' Phelo countered. 'How many procedures do you reckon we've done?'

'Thousands,' we all said at the same time.

'Think you'll miss this place?' I asked. 'It's been bonkers and wild, but ... maybe ... fun at times?'

'Ja,' said Kobus. 'I'll miss some things but not others. The things I wanted to remember, I think I forgot ... and the stuff I wanted to forget, I still remember.'

'I'm looking forward to having some time back. I've heard comm serv isn't as hectic as internship,' I said. 'It also pays a bit better ...'

'Ja, time to focus on some personal stuff. I've given enough time to this hospital,' said Kobus.

'Anything specific?' I asked.

'I want to run the Comrades Marathon.'

'With all those ciggies you smoke? Come, wena,' said Phelo.

'No, I'm serious! I'm putting these down and getting back in shape. I haven't eaten or exercised properly in two years and it's time to get back to it. Come join me!'

'Never! I'm not crazy!' laughed Phelo. 'Who in their right minds runs ninety kilometres? Insanity ...'

'What about you, Al? Wanna run it?'

'God, I don't think so, Kobus. I did a 21K at varsity and nearly died. Ninety seems too far. I'll cheer you on, though.'

There was a pause.

'I don't regret my time here but I'm not sad to be saying goodbye. Al, you hang in there, take what you can and get out before it scars you,' said Kobus.

'Don't listen to him,' said Phelo. 'Don't let this place make you hard. You can do a lot of good here, but you need to block out the bullshit. Focus on the patients, not the crappy folk in charge.'

'What the actual hell?!' Our chat was interrupted by Anwar. 'They found it! Or ... they sort of did.'

'What are you talking about?' I asked.

'My car! Remember it got stolen when we were doing O and G? I finally managed to convince the hospital to access the CCTV footage. What a fucking nightmare, but that's another story. They finally sent it to me and take a look ...'

We watched a grainy black-and-white video on Anwar's phone. It was from a single camera outside the ophthalmology entrance. We saw Anwar's car, driven by two men. At the boom, the car came to a halt and the engine died (a security feature when the key wasn't in the ignition). A security guard diligently checked the boot and then waved them through disinterestedly. But the car wouldn't restart. We could see gesticulations and fretful waving from the thieves who were clearly worried their jig may have been up. One of them got out and had a word with security who then walked behind the car and helped the thieves push it through to the main road. Once through, the men waved in thanks and drove off.

'I can't believe it,' Anwar muttered. 'Security *helped* them? What the hell is the point of those booms if security is going to lay out the red carpet for thieves?'

'Inside job, or are security just idiots?' Kobus asked.

'I don't think we'll ever know,' said Anwar. 'With this hospital, either is equally possible ...'

For some extraordinary reason that seemed like the ideal note on which to bring internship at Chris Hani Baragwanath Hospital to its end.

PART 2
The History

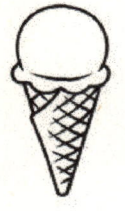

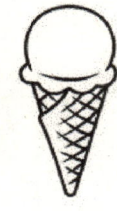

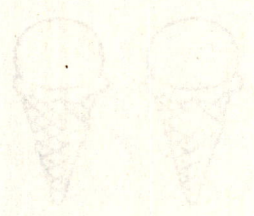

Chapter 9
POWERLESS

Something was different from that very first drink. I was seventeen years old and had decided to officially 'get drunk' with a friend. This was the first time we had ever had a drink and we decided we were going to do it properly.

The evening started out inauspiciously. We had tried to hit one of the trendy clubs in Rosebank but our excuses about 'lost IDs' didn't sway the hulking bouncers who waved us away in irritation for being underage. Deflated, we returned to my house and promptly raided my parents' liquor cabinet. What we lacked in drinking experience we made up for with a steely determination to get as wasted as we possibly could. We tried a bit of everything – gin, whisky, vodka, beer – much to the amusement of my younger brother, who egged us on by feeding us ever-more revolting concoctions.

We drank far too much, far too quickly, and I ended up passing out on the slightly damp front lawn before being helped to my bed by my mother. The memories of that night are hazy, but the memories of the *feeling* are crystal clear.

To this day, I can still taste the harsh bite of the whisky coating my tongue. I can feel the shocking burn as the vodka sent my salivary glands into overdrive, before smashing into the back of my throat and hurtling down into my stomach. I remember the warmth that enveloped me when the alcohol entered my bloodstream. It started somewhere deep inside; a glow that extended from my abdomen and radiated outwards, leaving what felt like delicious humming fragments scattered throughout my body. The world may have become unsteady, but the relief from the anxieties nestled in my brain was as solid as granite. My breathing gradually became deeper. My thoughts, which were previously sloshing around in my brain, quickly emptied, like a burst inflatable pool. For the first time, I felt unperturbed by the anxieties of school, the need to be smart, my looks, my kinky hair, and how generally uncool I was. For just a few hours, while the alcohol coursed hotly through my veins, it was as if a treasured childhood blanket had been thrown over me, smothering my fears, shielding me from the barbs and jabs of typical teenage life. It wasn't that the alcohol made my problems go away; rather, it was that it made me feel like they didn't matter.

Once, after a minor episode of bullying in my prep-school years, and as part of their initial assessment, I had been asked by a counsellor what I wanted more than anything else in the world. 'To take a girl to the movies, sir. And for her to hold my hand,' was my reply. This modest answer belied the fact that, at that time, I was in *no* danger of having my hand romantically held by anyone. I was an academic and studious boy with bad skin and thick, wavy hair that I hated. Like many introspective and academic teens, I thought scholastic achievement was overrated. I would have traded every History and English award I ever won for popularity with my peers and success with the opposite sex. My self-worth at the time was built around 'being smart' and since I was in no way physically imposing, it was my only armour against the cruel jibes of adolescence. I realised that my wits were a weapon, too. Like a scorpion, I could wound before I could be wounded, but it occasionally resulted in a relatively harmless punch to the gut from a wounded peer, which is what led me to the counsellor and the remark about girls and movies.

Since my identity was carved and moulded around my brain's ability to out-think any of life's problems, it simply never occurred to me what might happen when the problem *was* my brain. And what might happen when I could no longer rely on it to get me out of a tricky predicament.

A palisade wall of intelligence can take years to erect but can be brought down, Jenga-style, by a single brick of ridicule. Throughout my teenage years, to protect myself, I realised that, at all costs, I needed to avoid being made to look foolish. This desire to constantly succeed drove me with a wild but occasionally directionless force. It also created a slightly false sense of bravado because to avoid compromising comments, I frequently had to lie. I quickly realised that people were more likely to believe a confidently stated falsehood than a quietly whispered truth.

As an academic teen, I was given significant responsibility, on top of a number of extracurricular activities. My achievements accumulated but I frequently felt like a juggler, forced to keep too many balls in the air. From afar it appeared I was managing, but internally the effort of maintaining competence in so many fields was utterly wearying. And so, when that alcohol hit my bloodstream, even for a brief period, I was primed for that weariness to be lifted. And when it was, I was elated. It was a sensation I didn't fully understand at the time, but I knew I wanted – *needed* – to experience it again.

It's a cliché that things happen slowly until they don't, but it applied strongly to my early drinking days. While it was mostly manageable during that final school year, even then some serious red flags were raised.

By winter, I already had a bottle of my parents' whisky stowed away in my cupboard. I'd take a few swigs before going to a party for some 'Dutch courage'. For a while those few sips suited me. I found the liquid courage helped to lubricate potentially friction-filled interactions, and I loved the slightly off-kilter perspective it gave me.

My second major blackout, after that first night at home, occurred a few months later.

My friends and I were going to a big, end-of-term party at a schoolmate's fancy house in the jacaranda-studded suburbs of Johannesburg. With the term completed, and the prospect of a month's holiday ahead of us, I didn't see any reason to hold back. Some pre-party drinking was common, and a group of friends congregated at my house. Everyone was enjoying a beer or three, but I felt I needed an additional buzz, so I secretly started sneaking off to my room and taking swigs from the hidden whisky bottle. One sip felt good, four felt better, so I kept going. Suddenly, like a quick cut in a movie, I found myself at the party. The memories are scattered, but I recall a desperate urge to find the bar to get more drinks. I remember nearly getting into a fight after bumping into someone and spilling his drink. I remember my heavy breathing and thinking that the lights in the house and the darkness of the night were a strange mix. I remember stumbling out. And then, the next thing I knew, I woke up at the bottom of the garden at 3am, the house dark and deserted.

Due to a misunderstanding (and having a good mate also called Alastair), two sets of friends thought I had caught a lift home with the other. I didn't own a cellphone at the time and the host had locked up and gone to stay with his girlfriend. Everything was dark. Everyone had left. No one was looking for me or waiting up. I was cold and shivering and still very drunk. It was too cold to wait until the sun came up and I desperately wanted my bed. I climbed gingerly over the wall and headed in the approximate direction of my house.

I'm still not sure how I made my way home, but I managed to identify a few streets I knew, and followed them until I could see a familiar landmark. I'd repeat this tactic until I was close to my address. For some reason, ringing someone's doorbell and asking if I could use their phone never occurred to me. Or perhaps it did, but I was too embarrassed.

A well-dressed white kid staggering alone through some very dodgy parts of downtown Johannesburg was an inviting target for muggers or thugs, but, amazingly, I was left in peace, and three hours later I stumbled into the house. My parents, when they heard the story, were so relieved that I had made it back in one piece that I wasn't even heavily punished. But the habit of wandering off alone while wasted would get me into serious trouble over the years to come.

Episodes like this became more and more frequent but were masked by the heavy drinking culture of early university years. While I was able to maintain my academic performance in my first year of medical school, my grades began to suffer in the second. Too frequently, I would be hungover at morning lectures, staring morosely at a cup of instant coffee instead of listening to complex human physiology. When it came to dissecting our cadaver to learn about anatomy, the nausea after a heavy night of drinking, combined with a throbbing headache and the inescapable stench of formaldehyde, made retaining the complicated Latin names of tiny muscles and nerves extremely difficult. I slipped from being near the top of the class in first year to nearly failing my first anatomy test in my second.

Whenever I went out with my friends, I drank to get drunk, seeking an imaginary line where I could *feel* the effects of intoxication without *appearing* overly drunk. It was a line I searched for with impressive industry, but never found. I subsequently discovered that this is because it doesn't exist. In my mind, I always needed just a bit more to reach the ideal state of drunkenness, but would then wake up the next morning having overshot it completely and behaved embarrassingly. In my eyes I was never drunk enough, whereas in my friends' I had always overdone it. Often, I would be reminded of people I had met, conversations I had had, or inappropriate things I had done, of which I had little or no recollection whatsoever. I would either have to bluff my way through, or concede that I had just had a 'big one' and try to laugh it off. It was here that my ability to lie, honed in high school, came to my aid. But no amount of bravado could hide a truth that was rapidly emerging: I was an ugly drunk. Some people believe that alcohol doesn't change your personality and that, like a Russian doll being opened, it merely reveals a deeper version of who you really are. If that is the case, the image revealed me as someone who was argumentative, ill-tempered and unyielding. Like a planet with its gravitational pull reversed, when I was drunk people drifted away from me. I began to feel lonelier and lonelier, which only spurred the drinking on.

When, after two years at university and two years in residence, it came time to move to outside accommodation, none of my extremely close group of school friends wanted to live with me. Constant drinking meant that I had also failed to forge many new friendships while in residence. It was a gut punch. I convinced myself that it was because of some imagined vendetta or callousness on their part. The truth was they didn't want to be around me when I drank.

The anger at being excluded was wounding and, like a bleeding animal, I lashed out, turning an external disappointment into internal self-loathing. I was trapped in a cycle of wanting to show my friends I could be independent of them, while desperately wanting their approval and acceptance. I eventually managed to find an old school acquaintance to live with, but it was not the scenario I had imagined when my friends and I were excitedly planning life with each other outside of UCT accommodation.

As third year progressed, my peers put their immature ways and heavy drinking behind them and began focusing on their studies. With fewer parties happening, there were stretches of time when people I knew were not drinking at all. This was shockingly distressing. I remember one night standing in the shower and feeling panicked because it was a Wednesday, and the next excuse to drink was a twenty-first birthday party on the Saturday. This four-day stretch felt like an intolerably long time to be without the warmth I craved, and I remember shivering with anxiety despite the warm water cascading down me.

In response, my solitary drinking escalated. Which is when the wheels really started to fall off. One year later, I found myself in a psychiatric and rehabilitation hospital for depression and alcohol abuse.

We've all read stories, or watched movies, about the desperate lengths that substance abusers will go to in pursuit of their fix. My story is as banal as it is common, if no less tragic. I simply spent long periods of time, alone, drinking to get drunk.

As with any addiction, my drinking escalated, consuming my life in the process. In Afrikaans the word for a substance abuser is 'verslaafde', which means 'slave'. This is a vivid and appropriate word. Not only did my addiction rob me of everything I held dear, but it also perversely managed to convince me that the substance I was abusing was the only thing I could rely upon to make me feel better.

Many people have the odd glass of wine, or beer, by themselves. Repeatedly drinking, alone, for the purpose of getting drunk, is the domain of the person living with alcoholism. But even then, a level of denial, particularly to myself, was required. This manifested in how I bought and stored alcohol. The 'logical' thing to do would have been to buy a few half-jacks of vodka and many bottles of cheap wine, and store them in my cupboard. This is the tactic I initially tried, but it failed for two reasons.

Firstly, the alcohol never lasted as long as it was supposed to. Whatever booze was in the house would be drunk, and fairly quickly at that. This included alcohol that belonged to my digs' mate. She would sometimes leave a half-drunk bottle of wine in the fridge (this was an alien concept to me, like those people who can eat half a bar of chocolate and then put the rest away). I would inevitably drink the bottles of wine and then try to come up with excuses as to what had happened to them. Some of my tales were incredibly lame. I would say I had knocked the bottle over while reaching for something else, or that I had had guests over who must have helped themselves. No one was buying this nonsense. But I learned that to avoid going completely overboard, I had to limit the amount of alcohol around me.

Secondly, and more importantly, maintaining the illusion in my own mind that I didn't have a problem was difficult with a cupboard full of booze. The ridiculousness of my narrative confronted me every time I stared at the shelves packed with bottles, pricking my conscience with the unwelcome thought that *this wasn't normal*. Whereas, if alcohol was bought spontaneously, this could all be avoided. The only sticky issue was procuring it.

I quickly learned where all the nearby bottle stores were, but in an effort not to appear to be too much of a 'regular' at any of them, I rotated my patronage. So if I went to Wholesale Liquor on Monday, I'd go to Barney's Bottle Store on Tuesday, and then buy a few bottles of white wine when I went to Woolworths on Wednesday.

This constant toing and froing between various liquor stores was both time-consuming and exhausting. I remember the feeling of terror of rushing to get to a bottle store on a Saturday before sales closed at 5pm. The beating heart, the cursing at every red light, the honking at motorists driving too slowly, the barely concealed panic at the thought of being without alcohol until Monday, and the massive rush of relief at arriving at 4:59pm and charging in as the rail was being put around the alcohol and grabbing a precious bottle. I remember, too, the feeling of despair at arriving a few minutes late and having to bargain with the owner, placatory cash hastily shifted under the counter.

By the middle of third year, I knew which stores were 'flexible' with their sales. Of course, I wasn't the only one making a last-gasp effort at buying alcohol, and I recall standing in line, trying not to make eye contact with the people around me, all of us nursing the bottles of alcohol in our hands like religious artefacts.

There came a point when the buying of alcohol itself became part of the routine. I would feel the bite in the back of my throat while walking to the store; the anticipation levels rising. On entering, the sights and smells overwhelmed me, immediately saturating all my senses.

The bottles gleaming on the shelves, the acrid smell of alcohol, the whirr of the refrigerators keeping things cool, the tease of the bottles as I ran my hands over them, caressing them with reverence.

I'd pause and savour what was coming, my whole body becoming soft, like clay. I took my time, pretending that I was deciding what to buy before nonchalantly going to the vodka section. Only one decision really needed to be made: a half-jack or a full bottle. By this stage, drinking beer alone was not a regular occurrence because it was simply too much hassle. I'd have to drink at least four beers before I felt anything, and I'd then have to constantly go to the bathroom to pee. The same effect could be attained with a couple of swigs of neat vodka. It was a no-brainer.

I knew that a half-jack would probably do the trick, but my tolerance had slowly increased. A half-jack was no longer getting me to the level of inebriation I desired so I had started buying a full bottle. Earlier in the week, I had drunk about three quarters of a bottle and found myself overly wasted and blacking out. Also, not ideal. So, the perfect amount was probably two-thirds. A whole bottle was too much but I would probably drink it anyway. If I bought a half-jack, I might be left unsatisfied. In the end, I'd compromise and buy a half-jack and a bottle of cheap wine.

I generally waited to get to my bedroom before cracking the cap, catching the first whiff of the deliciously noxious smell, then putting the bottle to my lips. Sometimes, however, I couldn't endure the wait till I got home. I'd pop into a public bathroom to have a few swigs. The flickering, cheap fluorescent lights and filthy floors, which I ordinarily found repulsive, I tolerated because I needed my fix.

I was trapped in a situation where I couldn't admit to anyone how much I was drinking. My girlfriend at the time started expressing concerns about how my behaviour was impacting our relationship. I promised her that I would cut down, but the thought of staying over at her house for an entire weekend where my alcohol use would be closely observed was too much to bear, and I'd smuggle in a bottle of vodka and hide it in one of her cupboards when she wasn't looking.

My family and friends were expressing concerns, too. I'd promise them (sincerely) that I would cut down or stop drinking altogether. I'd throw all my alcohol away and swear that I wouldn't drink any more, but my good intentions usually lasted a week at the longest, and usually much shorter than that. Instead of pouring my energy into my studies, or my relationships, or my partner, it went into the procuring, using and hiding of alcohol. It therefore wasn't surprising that all my relationships began to suffer.

Addiction is an exercise in constantly adjusting the invisible line of acceptability. People say, 'I could never drink neat vodka on my own,' but they don't realise that people with alcoholism don't jump from social drinking to mixing whisky with their cornflakes overnight. Addiction, rather, is a process that goes at different speeds and in different increments for different people. You find a marker and repeatedly tell yourself and others that you will go this far and no further. But soon you find yourself nudging that line again and again until eventually you simply cross it and move it to a new position. For me, no drinking during the week became no drinking on Monday or Tuesday, became no drinking before 5pm, became no drinking before 12pm, became no vodka for breakfast. Because the process was gradual, the insanity of having an internal debate about whether it was normal to be holding out till 9am to have a drink simply didn't register. The line had shifted imperceptibly until it had vanished altogether.

By the end of third year, I was barely able to hold things together. I had managed, with gritted teeth, to scrape a period of sobriety together to push through the end-of-year exams. When they were finished, a fatigue I had never felt before descended on me. Every muscle fibre in my body was weary. Initially, I thought that it was the stress of the exams. More likely it was simply the intense physical and emotional energy I had expended on white-knuckling my way through sobriety while heavily addicted.

That holiday my girlfriend's father was tragically murdered on his farm during the unrest in Zimbabwe. I had to leave my holiday in the Eastern Cape to fly to Zimbabwe to be with her. At the airport, I bought two bottles of vodka.

Instead of supporting my girlfriend through a terrible personal tragedy, I used the sadness of the occasion as an excuse to get drunk instead. While I may have been physically present for the funeral and the aftermath, emotionally, I couldn't have been further away. She dumped me shortly thereafter in an act of sanity that I simply could not see at the time.

I had loved her very deeply, but gradually my drinking had turned my focus away from her and all my attention became concentrated on my next drink. The personal tragedy was the final straw, but in reality, while I was drinking, I was not a good boyfriend. This truth was too much to bear, and instead of facing it, I blamed her. I then used my anger as grist to the mill of my resentment, which ultimately fuelled my addiction.

There is no lonelier a disease than addiction. It's a loneliness that gnaws at the soul. The loneliness of being deeply and irrevocably cut off from other human beings. Like jumping into icy water, the shock of being so isolated often left me gasping in despair. I'd sometimes lie on my bed at night and scroll through the numbers on my phone, believing that there was not a single person I thought I could call. Misery, loneliness, anger and self-pity clashed every day, duelling until there was a victor. The winner then provided me with more than enough justification to keep drinking.

I didn't give my ex-partner the space that she needed to heal and would often get drunk and send her ugly texts, trying to make her feel guilty for dumping me. She initially responded with concern, and then distress. When she realised it was the alcohol talking, she ignored me. One night, in a rage of self-pity, I went to her apartment and kept my finger on the buzzer to try to get her to speak to me. Her roommate came down and told me firmly to scram, but I stayed put and continued ringing the buzzer. In desperation, she called my friends, who eventually arrived and dragged me away. I was subsequently told she had almost called the police.

The situation became unsustainable, and despite pleas from family and friends, warnings from the medical school, and appointments with psychologists and psychiatrists, I was unable to stop drinking. My friends became so worried about the constant smell of alcohol on me, the rumpled clothes, the dishevelled hair and the profound depression, that eventually I was summoned to a disciplinary meeting where my worst nightmare was confirmed: I was suspended from medical school until further notice. I'd have to go into a rehabilitation programme, and only upon successful completion of this programme, and maintenance of solid sobriety, would I be considered eligible to return.

My life as I knew it lay in tatters. The drinking had adversely affected my health and I looked wan and dejected. My sallow, pale face was contorted by misery and alcohol, and in the mornings I noticed the emergence of broken blood vessels on my nose, usually only seen in hardened drinkers in their later years. I have only seen my stoic, conservative father cry once, and that was when he flew down to Cape Town and saw what had become of his beloved, talented son. A young man, with every privilege and advantage, inexplicably squandering his life on cheap, sickly wine and bottles of pungent vodka.

PART 2: THE HISTORY

At the age of twenty-one, I was a hardened alcoholic. I just didn't know it yet.

In the days following my suspension, I visited several psychiatrists and recovery facilities. To deal with the stress, I'd usually drink before these visits. I settled on one of the fancier private rehabs in Cape Town. Nestled in the heart of suburbia, dappled by the light let in by large, shady trees, the rehab – at least superficially – had an aura of peace and tranquillity.

It was divided into two main areas: the psychiatric hospital, where patients with needs that required inpatient care were housed, and the rehabilitation unit, where I would be going.

I arrived on an uncharacteristically cold April morning. The sun shone without any warmth and the air was tinged with a wintery chill. I was ushered into a station for 'processing' where a medical history was taken by a stern nurse, and blood tests done to make sure I didn't have any glaring medical issues.

The inside of the building was clean, but with the air of a well-worn, lived-in space, not a harsh, sterile one. It was well heated; the warmth on the inside in sharp contrast to the cold I had walked through in the parking area. The walls were adorned with framed pictures of the twelve steps of Alcoholics Anonymous, or newspaper clippings of previous patients who had 'beaten addiction' and were now living happy, productive lives. In one, there was an interview with Eric Clapton, where he listed finding and maintaining sobriety as his greatest achievement. In another, Anthony Hopkins spoke about how achieving sobriety decades before had saved his life.

Outside the office, there was a whiteboard with a list of first names written on it. I presumed these were the current patients. Next to each name was a comment. Alongside 'Bobby' was written 'Can the fighter surrender to win?' The name 'Joe' was accompanied by 'Captain Recovery?'. Before I could read any further, a voice yanked me back into the processing room.

'How much do you drink?'

'Uh ... like ... in a day? A week?'

'Whatever you think is the most accurate, Alastair.'

Shame coursed through my body. I couldn't tell the truth. I had decided that I would present myself as a young guy going through a tough time, probably depressed, who clearly overdid it sometimes, but didn't really deserve to be here. In that way, I could be out as soon as possible.

Not every day, I told her. Mostly beer and wine. Occasionally the hard stuff. Never in the mornings. Not often as a treatment for a hangover (the 'often' raised an eyebrow from the nurse, so I quickly moved on). Last blackout was a while back ... New Year, I believe? But don't we all overdo it on New Year? This is all probably a bit of an overreaction.

The admission nurse dutifully wrote everything down, all the while maintaining a completely neutral expression. I had no idea whether she believed me or not, and I was desperate for her to frown at how benign I was making everything sound. Surely this guy shouldn't be here?

After taking my phone and searching my bag, I was shown to my room. I would be sharing with two roommates who were currently in a group session. My formal programme would begin the next day. In the meantime, I was given a Valium to mitigate my sudden abstinence from alcohol. I protested that I didn't get those effects, that I was nowhere near the tremor stages. The nurse just smiled and held the tablet out to me. I took it and collapsed on the bed, my mind whirring.

As my lids began to feel heavy, I heard voices entering the room. Then shuffling and laughter.

'Check the new guy. He's young. Probably a first-timer.'

'Yeah, maybe. I remember my first time like it was fucking yesterday. I was older than him, though. Remember yours?'

'God, such a long time ago. I'm so fucking tired of rehabs. Anyway, let's get a smoke, yeah?'

As their footsteps shuffled out, and the door closed, I was pulled into a deep blue darkness.

At breakfast the next morning, I was extremely groggy. I had slept for sixteen hours but felt terrible, like there was a weight in my limbs. I had been woken for the morning meditation but was still so sleepy from the Valium that I could hardly remember it. The only thing that stuck in my brain was the prayer we used to close the session. Everyone held hands and solemnly intoned: 'God, grant me the serenity to accept the things I cannot change, the courage to change the things I can, and the wisdom to know the difference.'

I did not consider myself religious, or even particularly spiritual, but I liked those words – they sounded simple but true. They gave me some much-needed focus, so I held onto them while I followed everyone to breakfast.

In the dining hall, I made myself a small bowl of cornflakes, which was all that I could handle given the nausea I was experiencing. For the first time since waking up, I was finally able to look around at my fellow patients. They were mostly white, and the hum of different accents and languages told me that while some were South African, many were foreign: mostly German, Dutch or British.

The group appeared diverse: middle-aged women and ageing hippies with long, grey hair. Teenagers and awkwardly dressed men in slacks who looked like they were far more comfortable in suits. Young, incredibly thin women and heavily tattooed skinheads. I couldn't imagine another scenario where such a disparate group would be sitting together.

As I surveyed the room, a middle-aged guy with thinning hair slid into the chair opposite me. With a noticeable thud, he plonked a well-thumbed book with a grey cover down on the table, entitled simply *Just For Today*.

'Morning, Stephen!' he beamed to a guy who was walking past with his breakfast tray.

To a woman sitting a few tables to our right he called, 'Stacey! Thanks for clearing those chairs up after the meeting. You're a star.'

He had the relentlessly optimistic air of someone who read a lot of self-help books. He smiled at me and held out his hand for me to shake.

'Hey man. I'm Joe. I'm the group leader so it's my job to welcome you. From the board, I assume you're ... Alastair?'

'Yeah. Nice to meet you.'

His handshake was firm and he squeezed harder than he needed to. 'First time?'

'Excuse me?'

'First time in rehab? You have the look of the newcomer.'

'Oh, yeah. Yeah, it is. Is it that obvious?'

'Hey! Don't be embarrassed. No one here is in any position to judge. If I may ask, what was your drug of choice? No wait! Let me guess ...' He stared at me disconcertingly for a few seconds. 'Got it! Coke! I'll bet you were a cocaine fiend like me.'

'Actually, no. Alcohol.'

'Ohhh! An alkie! You should chat to Brian over there. He's one of the drinkers as well. From Holland.'

'Seems like a lot of foreigners.'

'Ja. Rehabs are big business, and the overseas guys, especially Europeans, have learned that flying okes out to South Africa, keeping them in rehab for six weeks, and flying them back is cheaper than a three-week stay in their home countries. It's an absolute gold mine and its mostly untapped. Once I get outta here, I plan to open my own. It's not difficult and there's little regulation ...'

Joe explained that patients weren't differentiated based on their substance of choice, so while there were other alcoholics, there were also those addicted to a wide variety of other substances. These ranged from the prosaic and legal (diet pills, benzodiazepines) to the illicit and, to my mind, exotic (heroin, crack cocaine, quaaludes). The only thing we all had in common was, as Joe put it, 'Being totally fucked. Trying to repair our broken lives.' I also discovered that many of us were battling dual diagnoses. Eating disorders, gambling addiction, sex addiction, depression, bipolar mood disorder and stuff I hadn't heard of like 'co-dependency'. 'We're all fucking *mal*!' he chuckled. 'But at least we're around our own people.'

'I suppose,' I responded.

'Listen,' he said, putting a piece of bacon into his mouth, 'This programme *works*, okay? But you've got to surrender to it. Do what the counsellors tell you. Don't fuck around. Stay focused on your recovery and not the chicks. Get honest. It works if you work it, bru. There's no reason you can't be the fifteen per cent.'

'Fifteen per cent? What's that?'

'The percentage of people who find sobriety after rehab.' He shovelled another piece of bacon into his mouth.

'That doesn't sound great,' I murmured.

'Ja, addiction's a bugger. So make sure you start working the damn programme ASAP. If nothing changes, nothing changes.'

Tiring a little of the parade of slogans, I changed the subject. 'So how does it work here?' I asked.

'Every morning we get up early for meditation and the Serenity Prayer. Then it's breakfast, followed by lectures. After that, it's group sessions and then lunch. After lunch, it's life-story time and maybe some one-on-one stuff with your counsellor. Late afternoons are for art or relaxation. Dinner is early 'cos in the evenings an ex-patient comes and shares their story of recovery with us, or we go to meetings. The alkies go to Alcoholics Anonymous and the druggies like me go to Narcotics Anonymous. Which is a bit like AA, but with less God.'

He could see the frown I made at the mention of religion.

'Hey, listen. I can tell you're one of those intellectual atheist types. But that shit won't really fly here. You need to find *something* to believe in. It can be "God" or it can be the group, or the programme, or whatever, but if you think you're your own saviour, you'll be back in no time.'

'So what do you believe?' I asked.

'I try not to overthink it. I was raised a Christian, but I'm not sure I really buy all that Bible stuff. But I think God exists, so I just go with that.'

Before we could continue, he glanced at the clock on the wall. 'Shit, it's nearly lectures and we don't want to be late. Follow me.'

In my first set of lectures, I discovered that rehabs and recovery programmes in South Africa (including the one I was in) were primarily constructed around the Twelve-Step Program of Alcoholics Anonymous (AA), founded by Bill W. and Dr Bob in 1935. The tenets of the programme are as famous and worn as the well-thumbed copies of the *Big Book* (The AA 'Bible') used in thousands of meetings all over the world every day. AA's focus is primarily on the paradoxical benefit of 'one addict helping another' with the aim of working through the twelve steps sequentially. The steps themselves were treated with a reverence reserved for religious texts, with large posters scattered everywhere – attached to walls, hung in rooms, and emphasised via daily read-throughs. Slogans intrinsic to the programme were repeated over and over ('One day at a time', 'Turn it over', 'It works if you work it!', 'Don't quit five minutes before the miracle occurs', etc. etc.) Very basically, the purpose of the twenty-one-day stay was to get us detoxified off our drug(s) of choice, convince us to buy into the Twelve-Step Program, which included complete abstinence from all drugs and alcohol, and begin working the first few steps. Total abstinence was the goal. We were clearly unable to regulate our use and rehab was not about giving us tips and tricks to cut things down. Rather, it was hammered into us that it was only through abstinence that we would find freedom, and the *only* way to remain abstinent was through a rigorous practice of the Twelve-Step Program. This meant not just completing twenty-one days in rehab but maintaining ongoing connections through AA and NA meetings when we left.

Those early days still feel strange. I remember being confronted by Step 1: 'We admitted that we were powerless over our addiction – that our lives had become unmanageable' and feeling irritation. I had been able to think and reason my way out of every problem life had thrown at me so why would alcohol prove to be any different? If I could learn the minutiae of human anatomy, or the complexities of histopathology, surely I could find a way to moderate my drinking? What I needed was time and space; an opportunity to repair things with the people I had hurt. When I asked Joe what he made of Step 1, he responded, 'When most people have the first hit of the night, they know how things will end. When we have the first hit, it could go anywhere!' I could wrap my head around this and wanted to explore it further. Instead, I was being forced to attend 'P&D' (Powerless & Damages) groups. In these sessions, we were subdivided into groups of five or six. Everyone introduced themselves at the beginning of every group, followed by an acknowledgement that they were an addict or alcoholic. I remember saying the words, 'Hello, I'm Alastair, and I'm an alcoholic' and feeling somewhat benumbed. Had I sometimes drank alcoholically? Sure. Was I an alcoholic? I wasn't really convinced. I had seen alcoholics on the streets and in movies and they weren't like me.

The stated purpose of these groups was 'denial busting', with patients recounting the terrible toil the pursuit and use of their drug of choice had had on our lives. The aim was to show that we had little to no control over our drug of choice, and the terrible consequences that resulted from this. We were gently, but firmly, encouraged to be as honest as possible about our experiences. 'Sunlight is the best disinfectant' was a phrase that was frequently uttered.

The stories themselves ranged from the banal to the horrifying. Everything from forgotten anniversaries to serious suicide attempts. Joe recounted how, out of all the terrible experiences his addiction had exposed him to, the one that hurt the most was missing his daughter's fifth birthday because he was coked up in a strip club. He had sworn to her on everything he held dear that he would be there, but the pull of his addiction had simply been too strong.

The spectre of death was not far away in many of the experiences, and tales of overdose, hospitalisation and incarceration were all too common. The underlying thread that stitched all these together was a profound sense of isolation. Nothing was as important as getting that fix, but the attainment of that fix cut us off from the human connection that could have saved us. Somewhere, at some indefinable point, we had all become unmoored from the bonds with our friends and family. This had led to a profound spiritual loneliness, which only served as fuel for addiction.

I was fascinated and taken aback that people were so willing to reveal their souls and their shame, but I also realised I could never bare mine. The things I had done were so beyond the pale that if anyone found out, I would be irrevocably shunned. And I certainly would be barred from re-entering medical school. Besides, even the origin of my addiction was shameful. While many spoke about abuse and trauma that undoubtedly ignited and fed their addictions, I had no such excuse. I had had a privileged, middle-class upbringing, with an imperfect but loving family and supportive friends. I had wanted for nothing. Other than a brief spell of bullying at school, I had faced no real hardships or obstacles to success.

The trope of the damaged human, broken by life and circumstance, seeking solace in mind-altering chemicals is one that is deeply embedded in the common psyche. We understand and sympathise with this image. Who, on the other hand, would feel anything for the high-flying, wealthy white kid who drank excessively because … well … because of no reason that made sense? I definitely wouldn't show any mercy to such weakness. I'd tell him what a miserable waste he was; that he should get his shit together immediately. Thinking about it just made me angrier and more perplexed. As a result, after a few days, I began to look forward to the P&D sessions.

I found it comforting to nestle in the misery of the group as it enabled me to not have to think about my own shame. I could nod and 'empathise' and offer gentle solicitude while throwing around some of the lingo I was gradually acquiring. But I certainly wasn't about to open up about my own behaviour. The members in our group didn't need to know about the awful loneliness, the debasing drives to shebeens and bottle stores to buy the cheapest liquor imaginable, the endless lying, the retching in the middle of the night, the seedy infidelity, the time lost crying in self-pity. How would I have justified this? How could I tell them that what I really wanted was to learn to drink successfully? I simply couldn't fathom a life of sobriety, but in a group where abstinence was the only option,

I didn't feel I could voice my plan to take another route.

I was smart enough to know that I couldn't stay silent. The dynamics of the group ebbed and flowed on the tides of participation, and it was demanded that I contribute. As a result, I carefully tailored my 'powerless and damages' stories to be serious enough to justify bringing them up, but vague enough that no deeper truths were unearthed. I also decided to get the counsellors on my side.

I made sure I was on time for all group meetings, even the eye-rubbingly early ones. When we went to AA meetings, I would be the first to get into the shuttle, and the first to contribute. I'd help with setting up chairs and tidying up. My assignments were neat and punctual. I decided I would not provide the counsellors with any reason to keep me in that godforsaken spot for a day longer than necessary. At the end of my tenth day, on the large whiteboard, a comment was written next to my name by one of the counsellors. I eagerly went to read it, looking for the affirmation I believed I deserved; a sign that I was winning at this rehab game. Next to my name was written 'Captain Recovery? Time to get real?'.

This was the same message I had seen next to Joe's name the day I arrived. This time, it made me furious. I kicked the board down when no one was looking.

Almost everyone in rehab smoked. I was an occasional smoker (usually able to resist the urge except when I drank), but the smoke breaks at rehab do not exist to just satisfy the nicotine urges of fractious addicts. They are a crucial socialising event; a nexus where everyone gets together to unwind, debrief and gossip about counsellors or other patients. Coffee and intrigue were both plentiful.

I was irritated by the 'Captain Recovery' comment and in a stormy mood. I was sitting and smoking alone when I felt a presence next to me. It was Chad, a young guy of seventeen. He had been admitted a week after me after his parents found him sprawled outside the house, his body coursing with alcohol and crack cocaine.

He had maintained an aloof coolness throughout the early days, and it was obvious he had no real intention of changing his behaviour. His comment on the board had been 'If nothing changes, nothing changes'. On the one hand, I admired his honesty; unlike so many others there, he was resolutely unflinching in his rejection of a programme designed to convince him to adopt lifelong abstinence. On the other hand, I was irritated because his refusal to comply highlighted how desperate and disingenuous my own platitudes and actions were. His honesty showed up my own superficial efforts.

I turned to face him and noticed he had a smirk on his face, which seemed locked on me.

'Something funny, dude?' I asked.

'Nah. I just know a bullshitter when I see one.'

'What?'

'This school-prefect shit. It's so lame. Why are you pretending to play their game? I can see you don't buy it.'

'Some of us want to get out. Doing what they want is the fastest way. Fucking around just means more hassles and potentially more rehab. Is that what you want?'

He inhaled, seemed to give my words more thought than they deserved, flicked his ash, and said, 'Bru, I'm just keeping it real. This fucking place is telling me I can never have a single beer ever again? Not even one? I'm seventeen ... think I'm going to go through my twenties partying on water? No fucking way.' He grinned. 'But I've noticed you, Mr Prefect. You think you don't belong here. You think you can trick everyone. Saying all the right things; cosying up to the counsellors. At least I'm honest enough to not pretend I'm into it.' He flicked his cigarette away. 'They don't buy it, by the way. They know you're full of shit.'

'I'm trying my best.'

He laughed loudly. 'Ja? I saw the look in your eye when Damian was discussing his last binge. I saw the hunger. You're not done.' He lit another cigarette.

'Didn't realise you were an expert.'

'When this is your fourth go-round, you learn who's taking things seriously and who's not. You also get a good sense about who's going to make it.'

'So, an addictions expert *and* a fortune-teller? I'm impressed.'

'Nah, it's just numbers and common sense. I've been here enough times to know that quitting, and staying quit, is *hard*. Most of the folks here? They're not ready. Three weeks of groups and meetings isn't going to change that. You're *definitely* not ready.'

'So who is? Joseph?' I pointed to the middle-aged hippie from Germany with shoulder-length grey hair. I had picked him out at random but he seemed to be making good progress and was due to leave soon.

'Joseph? Who're you trying to kid? He managed to smuggle some hash inside his matchbox. Notice how he's always so happy in the evenings?' Now that he mentioned it, Joseph did seem to have a goofy grin on his face. 'Dude's too old. Set in his ways.'

'What about Olivia over there? If she doesn't get sober, she's losing her marriage and possibly her kids. Surely she's ready?'

'Olivia is fucking Don.' He glanced at the handsome thirty-something guy who had arrived a few days before. 'No way can she save her marriage. Her husband is the whole fucking reason she drinks in the first place. Drinking? Having sex with other dudes? It's all about getting his attention back.'

'You make it seem like addiction is some kind of choice. That's not what they tell us here. It's a disease.'

PART 2: THE HISTORY

He snorted, smoke venting through his nostrils. 'A disease? Nah. That's what we'd all *like* to believe. It makes us feel better. Makes it seem like all the fucked-up shit we did wasn't our fault. Powerless, right? Robots? Unable to resist?'

'Something like that ...' I murmured, thinking back to that morning's lecture about how once an addict picks up their substance of choice, they have no control over how much of it they will ultimately consume.

'Bullshit. If I got you drunk and then put another shot of vodka in front of you, but held a gun to your head and told you that if you drink it I'll blow your brains out, think you'd be able to resist?'

'I mean, that's a stupid scenario,' I said.

'Indulge me.'

'Okay. I guess so ...'

'Exactly! You *do* have power. You *do* have agency. Once you realise that, this whole charade and "kumbaya" crap falls apart. We're not sick. We just went through some shit that makes us want to forget. But once we deal with it, then we should be okay. My dad – hectic alkie. Drank a bottle of Johnnie Walker every day with lunch. But it was because he was unhappy at his job. Once he quit and started doing what he loved, he didn't need to drink any more. Easy. None of this rehab crap.'

'So why are you here? If it's all a choice and you could just stop, you would be spending your eighteenth year partying with friends, not in a fucking rehab. For – what? – the fourth time. Why do you keep drinking?'

He smiled. 'That is not something I'm going to share with a Captain Recovery.' He disappeared off to the dining hall.

I tried to forget the conversation, but it kept buzzing in my head. What Chad said made a lot of sense. I was drinking because I was unhappy. Possibly depressed. I needed to deal with the source of my unhappiness, and the excessive alcohol use would normalise. If I could get back to med school, convince my girlfriend to take me back, then I should be able to resist the booze. I could find a way. I just needed to get out.

'Don't listen to Chad.' It was Joe. He was leaving the next day and I congratulated him on making it through. I told him I was jealous because he was going home to his middle-class life with a loving wife and kids. 'He's young and angry. Young people don't want to be told they're not in charge of their lives. Truly admitting he has a problem would require him to take a long, hard look in the mirror and ask for help. He's not there yet. He hasn't hit rock bottom. But eventually his addiction will force his hand.'

I told him about the gun thing, about how we likely did have choice and agency.

'That's overly simplistic and Chad knows it. A decision made at the barrel of a gun is not a true decision. If it were simply a matter of deciding to stop, why would any of us be here? We would've stopped ages ago. Unless you think I don't love my daughter and wanted to miss her party? Or that you wanted to be kicked out of med school?'

I shook my head.

'It's complicated, man. But there's probably a reason you spend so much time worrying what it is instead of how to get better.'

'I just want to understand.'

'Focus on getting better instead.'

I settled into a routine of groups and one-on-one sessions with my counsellor. While many of the staff who worked there were recovering addicts, mine was not. Her name was Megan and she seemed suspicious of my behaviour, despite my best efforts to convince her otherwise. Towards the end of the three weeks, she called me for a private meeting.

'Alastair, while the team thinks you have made some progress, we have … concerns. We think it would be best if your recovery was continued in a safe, yet monitored environment, so we recommend that you go to a secondary facility for a few months.'

I had been expecting this, but it was still an unpleasant jolt. Chatter within the rehab confirmed that, generally, the counsellors recommended patients go into a step-down (or 'secondary') facility before being released into the big wide world again. A secondary facility provided a lot more freedom than the primary one I was in, but it was a far cry from being able to resume my regular life. I also knew that I was likely to spend at least another month (and likely more) there. The thought of more time in a rehab was an excruciating one, and I had secretly been hoping that my model behaviour would allow me the equivalent of 'skipping' secondary. Megan's words dashed those hopes. The medical school was also being evasive as to whether I could go back to resume my studies. With every day that their decision was delayed, the chances of returning to medical school that year diminished.

A blackness settled over my brain and a biting sensation returned to the tip of my tongue. What more could I do? What more did they want? I had turned my entire life upside down and it *still* wasn't enough? I had to spend even *more* time doing rehab?

'What do you think about that? Are you willing?' Megan's words brought me thudding back to my reality.

This question was a trap and we both knew it; a game that needed to be played even though both sides knew how it would ultimately end. If I answered 'No, I'm unwilling to go,' Megan would have responded, 'Clearly you still have a lot of self-will driving your life. This is anathema to the programme, which asks you to surrender yourself to a higher power. You have more work to do and you need to go to secondary.'

If I had responded, 'Sure, I'm willing,' Megan would have responded, 'Wonderful! I'm so glad you're amenable to our suggestions. You will certainly benefit from extra time in a safe environment.'

In the end, I mumbled something and nodded.

The final week was a blur. I told my life story somewhere in there. It was a key moment for addicts in rehab: recounting our entire lives and what led us to where we were. I still had no idea why I drank so much nor was I convinced I was completely without agency. I recounted my childhood, exaggerating small events to give them an undeserved significance that explained my spiritual loneliness. I wrote about some of my drinking, but omitted the most awful episodes. When it was over, I was praised for my 'honesty and vulnerability'. I simply felt hollow.

I went to a lot of AA meetings that I don't remember. I wrote down a lot of stuff and did some step work. Mostly, I was counting the hours until I could leave. Yes, secondary wasn't ideal, but it was better than being here. Once out, I could try to resurrect things, in my own way.

My farewell was odd. Fellow patients said some obligatory nice things about my progress. Counsellors expressed some concerns, but wished me well on the next stage. I remember getting my phone back and frantically checking to see if my ex had sent any messages. She hadn't. On the way to the secondary, I stared glumly out the window of the car taking me there. Everything seemed the same. I was trapped and alone.

Chapter 10
TAKE TWO

Secondary rehab was in a two-storey house in Mowbray, a slightly seedier part of town. The lush trees that surrounded the primary rehab were replaced with concrete apartment blocks and noisy taxi ranks. The rooms were smaller, showing signs of decay. Paint was peeling off the walls in places, and a thin layer of dust had collected on the windows. Unlike primary care, it was not a hospital and had no medical staff. The idea behind secondary care is to provide a bridge between the intensity of inpatient care and being alone in the outside world. Many people with addiction have spent so long focusing on their drug of choice that they have forgotten the basics of how to live. Some never learned at all. Secondary care provides a safe environment for those in recovery to find their feet.

On my arrival, I met my new counsellor, Darren. A portly, serious-looking man in his mid-forties, he had pock-marked skin, grey hair and deep crows' feet around his eyes hinting at the life experiences that had aged him more rapidly than most. He brusquely shook my hand and welcomed me to the secondary rehab.

The rules of the facility, as explained to me by Darren, were straightforward: each housemate, primarily, had to stay clean and sober. This was non-negotiable and routine drug and alcohol testing would take place. Use of any mind-altering substance would result in immediate expulsion. But secondary care could also be used as a springboard to get re-established in a job, to learn new skills, or to complete an education.

We all had to stay at the facility every night and curfew was 10pm on weekdays and 11pm on weekends. Attending dinner at 6pm every day (except Sundays) was compulsory, and we were expected to prepare a meal for our housemates once a fortnight. We had to attend at least five AA or NA meetings a week, but these could be at times and locations of our choosing. House feedback sessions took place on Saturday mornings and were compulsory. Everyone was assigned a counsellor and Darren was to be mine.

'One of the benefits of secondary care is the degree of flexibility we offer. Some housemates work, some study, some just ... meander around, drinking coffee and smoking cigarettes. Although we don't encourage that. Unless you're working on yourself, you're not growing.'

He turned and looked at me with a wary intensity I found disquieting. I wanted to say something, but his gaze indicated that this was not the right time to talk. He was one of those people who felt no need to fill silences. In fact, he seemed to revel in the discomfort they caused, and after what felt like an age, he smiled tiredly and said, 'We only grow when things are uncomfortable. Don't you agree?'

'Uh ... sure. I guess.'

'No guessing here, Alastair,' he said enigmatically, before striding off.

I relished the initial freedom the facility provided. On my first afternoon, one of the housemates took me to the nearby supermarket to stock up on supplies I had missed while in primary rehab. I bought jelly beans, Coca-Cola and marshmallows. In the early stages of my recovery, I discovered that sugar took the edge off some of the cravings, and I planned to stock up. I also bought some deodorant, toothpaste and mouthwash.

On my way out, I noticed a bottle store next to the supermarket. This was my first sighting of anything alcohol-related since I had been admitted to rehab over three weeks ago. Immediately, a bitter, vinegary taste flooded my mouth. Saliva started coursing along the side of my tongue and I had to swallow to stop myself from drooling. I felt a bit dizzy and had to close my eyes and take a few deep breaths.

'It's always a bit of a shock.'

The comment from my housemate pulled me from my trance. 'What is?'

'Seeing your drug of choice for the first time after you've been in treatment. Nothing can really prepare you for it. Best thing is to acknowledge it and talk about it at a meeting later. You always feel better when you share this kind of stuff.'

'Thanks, I'll bear that in mind.'

I spat onto the pavement, took one last glance back, and then rejoined my companion on the walk back to the house. My breathing settled, the saliva stopped flowing, and when I got back I had a hot cup of tea to try to wash the metallic taste from my mouth. Like a permanent stain, however, nothing seemed to get rid of it. After a few hours, I welcomed the bitter bite it offered. I'd swirl my tongue around in my mouth and try recreating the same sensation that happened when I swigged that first mouthful of vodka. In response, my nerve endings came alive, the hairs on my arms pricked up and my breathing quickened.

I didn't talk about it at the meeting later.

The following day, I went for a walk along the river nearby. I lit a cigarette and watched the water gently flow by and thought about how I was going to return to my old life, but drink manageably. It wasn't going to be easy, but I knew that if I could just get through the next month, I'd be okay. In addition to going home and getting my girlfriend back, I could hopefully convince the relevant authorities at the university that I was worthy enough to be readmitted. I just needed to get out of here as quickly as possible. I would do what was asked of me – whatever it took to minimise the amount of time I had to stay.

I was filled with a renewed sense of hope and purpose. I *could* have my old life back. Some readjustments needed to be made regarding alcohol, but it was possible. What was a month anyway? I could see friends, go to a movie and even the regular meetings were becoming more bearable. Filled with a burst of energy, I saw a small pebble nearby and decided to try to skim it across the water. I picked it up and felt its smoothness against my fingers. Crouching low, I tried to flick my wrist to get it to skim. The arm motion felt great, my wrist flicked with a satisfying snap, and the pebble flew from my hand with momentum and speed. On the way, it clipped a reed, spun in the air, and crashed into the water with a graceless thud, before sinking to the bottom.

Later that week, I was irritable and restless. I was supposed to have a combined counselling session with my ex and, while it was ostensibly part of the ongoing denial-busting (she would lay out all the awful things I had done when I was drunk), I was secretly hoping to use it as an opportunity to show her I had changed. That I was reformed; different. Once she saw the effort I had made, she would take me back.

I was nervous the whole day before the session. I smoked cigarette after cigarette and paced anxiously back and forth. My head was whirring with ideas and emotions flew through my heart like purposeless ghosts. I needed something to distract me, maybe a sweet or a fizzy drink would help.

I told the counsellors I was heading up to the supermarket to buy a newspaper and other supplies and strolled up.

I bought what I wanted, but instead of walking home something strange happened. It felt automatic, like my legs were treading a well-worn path along a route that was comforting and routine. I approached the bottle store next to the supermarket, and the moment I entered that eye-wateringly sour taste settled on my tongue. This time I welcomed the bitter, acrid – but at the same time – comforting sensation.

I was surrounded by alcohol and it was dizzying. I was overcome with a sensation both comfortingly familiar and violently alien, like a loved one giving you a warm hug after admitting to a terrible betrayal. I felt my muscles tense up. I shouldn't be in here. ('Spend enough time in a barber shop and you're going to get a haircut,' was a meeting-acquired phrase that rang in my head.) But there was an illicit thrill, too.

By now, things were automatic. I wandered slowly along the aisles, my eyes savouring the bottles around me, drinking them in. I repeated the walk around the store three or four times, almost as if I was hoping to absorb the alcohol through osmosis.

Without thinking, I grabbed a half-jack of vodka and a bottle of Coke to mix it in. I didn't usually dilute or mix my drinks, but I needed something to store the vodka in that I could plausibly have in my room. I also hoped the Coke would disguise the odour of alcohol.

While paying, my bowels suddenly cramped and I desperately needed the bathroom. I dashed to the public toilet, which was as vile as you'd imagine one nestled in a busy bottle store would be. A single light dangled unsteadily from the roof, covered in a brown layer of god knows what. I retched into the basin, bringing up bile and saliva, and groaned as I relaxed on the fetid toilet seat. My body, it seemed, was cleansing itself in anticipation.

I suddenly thought about my parents. I thought about my dad and the tears running down his face when he saw what I had been reduced to a few weeks before. I thought about the friends who had so diligently and kindly visited me while I was in the rehab facility. I remembered their words of encouragement; their belief that I could get through this. I remembered my ex-girlfriend's face when I had got drunk before her father's funeral; the mixture of contempt and pity as I made slurred and inappropriate comments to the gathered mourners. I remember promising her that this wasn't who I was; that I would get better. I thought about being so desperate for a beer but not having any money, so I had drunk a cup of urine as payment. I remembered the guffaws of the guys who made me do it still echoing in my head, and I remembered promising myself I would never, ever feel that type of humiliation again. I thought about all these things and took a long, hard look in the mirror. I didn't know who it was staring back, but I knew he had courage. I knew he was better than this. I poured the vodka down the drain.

I splashed some water on my face and fled, leaving the booze behind.

When I arrived back at the rehab everyone could see I was shaken. Darren asked if I was okay, but I knew I couldn't tell my counsellor I had just been meandering around a bottle store and bought alcohol.

'Probably something I ate,' I mumbled. He looked unpersuaded.

'Have you been drinking?' The bluntness of his question took me by surprise.

'No! What? How could you say such a thing? Just not feeling great is all. Your dinner last night wasn't exactly a gourmet feast.' He let the jibe bounce off him.

'So if we were to give you a breathalyser test right now, you would pass?'

'Of course. Happy to do it any time.'

He looked unimpressed by my bravado, but decided not to test me.

'I'm worried about you, Alastair. You're keeping things from us. Shame and secrets are what drive this disease.'

'Don't worry about me, Darren. I'm good. In fact, I'm better than good. I managed to overcome quite a hurdle today. A challenge was put in front of me that I overcame. I'm quite proud of myself.'

'Want to talk about it?'

'Nah. But I stared down a demon today and it didn't get the better of me.'

He frowned. 'You don't beat Mike Tyson in the ring by outpunching him. You beat him by not getting in the ring in the first place.' He loved his aphorisms so much and I found myself getting irritated again. But fighting with counsellors wasn't going to get me released early so I nodded and walked away.

At the AA meeting that night, the whole group was ablaze with news of an ugly relapse. During the smoke breaks there was breathless chatter about someone who had shared their story the previous week, but it had subsequently been discovered he had been drunk at the time.

Gossip fuels early recovery, with stories of relapse acting as both a warning of the hazards of 'going back' as well as confirmation that someone else's recovery wasn't always as strong as we thought it was. Responses to relapses in the group ranged from 'I'm shocked! How could this have happened?!' to 'It was inevitable. He stopped seeing his sponsor ages ago. He was hanging out with drinking buddies. He was going back to the strip clubs. I saw this a mile away.'

Once the shock had worn off, the inevitable next question followed: How bad was it? There was an aura of salaciousness around this question. Perhaps it was because of a dislike of the person in question, or perhaps it was simple curiosity or concern. Most likely, it was a desire to experience, albeit fleetingly, the chaos of active addiction again, like an ex-smoker who wanders purposely through a cloud of cigarette smoke. The rush that only the constant oscillation between the highest of highs and lowest of lows can bring, a rush ironed smooth by the regular monotony of rehab, meetings and anti-depressants.

'Bad. He disappeared for a whole weekend, blew fifty grand on a stripper, then crashed his car into an idling truck. He's in the hospital now. Ruptured spleen.'

I cast my mind back to who had shared the previous week, and with a jolt, I recalled that it had been Joe, the group leader from the primary rehab, the original 'Captain Recovery' before I had assumed the mantle.

I was shocked. In rehab Joe had seemed to have it all together. He had been so positive and optimistic about the programme and his future. Upon leaving, he had the aura of someone who followed all the suggestions; he had found a sponsor (someone senior to you in the programme to help you work the steps); he was attending regular meetings; he shared openly and honestly about his struggles, while always maintaining a hopeful and optimistic air.

Now I heard that he had started drinking a few days after leaving rehab and had only come to meetings to convince his wife he was sober. He had apparently started gambling again and had blown R200 000 in one night at GrandWest Casino. Now he was broken in hospital.

I felt numb. If even the best of us were powerless against the ravages of this disease what was the point in struggling on? Was abstinence for a prolonged period even possible? Rehab seemed to be a merry-go-round of people with addiction jumping on and off again. The only ones who seemed to be winning were the owners of the rehabs, charging exorbitant rates.

Rather than joining in with the gossip, I walked off to spend some time by myself. I smoked another cigarette while everyone filed slowly back into the meeting for the second half. I didn't join them. I simply couldn't stomach any more slogans and platitudes, which ultimately didn't resonate with me. My mind was focused on the combined session with my ex the next day. She had needed a lot of persuasion to agree to come. After initially being reticent, she had only changed her mind when the counsellors told her they felt she would offer an invaluable perspective on the harm my drinking had caused. I was still hoping to use it as an opportunity to convince her to give me another chance, to show her I had changed. But I was anxious and couldn't stop shivering. This was my chance and I dare not blow it.

I watched the wispy smoke from my cigarette drift into the chilly evening air and waited for everyone to come out of the meeting.

The next morning, the day of the meeting with my ex, I didn't need to think about anything. There was no aimless ambling or meandering. After breakfast, I walked to the bottle store filled with purpose and determination. It felt so natural, as if my legs were strolling along a well-trodden path. I was being pulled but felt no inclination to resist. I got what I needed and in a flash was outside the shop again, feeling the weak sunshine on my face.

People shuffled past me, getting on with their day and hurrying to their jobs. There were jokes and smiles and small talk. I felt disconnected from every one of them.

I galloped into a second-hand bookstore and went to the bathroom. I poured half the Coke into the sink and topped it up with the vodka. The guilt and reservations of the previous day were gone, replaced with a numbing sense of resolve.

When it happened, there was relief. The relief that can only be felt by the beaten who give up when they know they never had a chance anyway. Relief that the punishment was over. There would be no more struggling. I had done it – I had relapsed. Now I just had to make sure no one found out.

I had intended to drink only a little, just to ease the nerves, but once the vodka entered my system, a calm washed over me and I craved more.

By the time I got back to the recovery house, I had drunk almost the whole bottle.

When I saw my ex, the first thing I noticed was that she had dyed her mousy brown hair a vivid shade of red. The second thing was that she looked extraordinarily beautiful, her hard edges given a hazy sheen by the alcohol. But the stern expression on her face told me that, to her, this meeting was purely business. She was here to say her piece and then leave. There would be no reunion today. My legs felt unsteady and my body was covered in an unhealthy layer of sweat from the warmth of the liquor in my body.

When the session started, she started by telling the counsellors what a challenge it had been to date me when I drank. How, as time went on, my addiction had filled the spaces of our relationship, nudging her further and further towards the periphery, until one day she realised she was tired of being a spectator. She was visibly angry at certain points, especially when she recounted how I had let her down when she needed me most – right after her father's death. She was neither unfair nor unkind; she was simply telling the story, experienced by millions of people every day, of someone finding themselves dating someone addicted to alcohol. I stared at the floor, kneading my fingers into each other, and searching my crashing, swirling brain for a response to the litany of failures she brought up. By the time she had finished, the room was spinning. I realised it was my turn to respond.

I immediately teared up and launched into a maudlin and rambling apology. I declared, for the thousandth time, how sorry I was, how much I missed her, how I wished she would give me another chance. It quickly became apparent that I was drunk; that the words coming out of my mouth were worse than meaningless; they were an insult. It was as if I was spitting in her face.

Darren could see something was wrong, quickly terminated the session and breathalysed me. I watched dejectedly as the yellow crystals turned pink in response to the alcohol on my breath. There it was in front of me – I was drunk.

The rest of the day collapsed. My things were packed up and I was sent straight back to primary rehab. All the way there, pathetic tears of self-pity streamed down my face. I had no idea what would happen next, nor did I particularly care. It felt as if I had lost everything important in my life and I was back to square one.

I was given another Valium on arrival and promptly went to bed. I slept through the rest of the day and most of the night. When I awoke, I initially had no idea where I was or why. For a few brief, blissful milliseconds, everything seemed all right. Then the headache pulsed through my brain with a nauseating ferocity and it all came back to me.

I was back to square one.

The time following my relapse is hidden beneath a miserable haze. I stayed at primary rehab while the counsellors decided what to do with me. Numbed on benzodiazepines, time seemed to ooze slowly like toothpaste out of a tube. As I was not a formal inpatient doing a programme, I was excluded from all the groups and counselling. I wandered around aimlessly, sensing the pitying looks from fellow patients who only a few days before had seen me leave on a triumphant note after completing the programme. The tut-tuts and I-saw-it-comings felt audible, even if they were never expressed out loud. Finally, I had a meeting with the head of the rehab.

'Alastair, you're a mess. I wish we could say we didn't see this coming, but that would be a lie. Most of us thought you'd be back; we just didn't think it would be so soon. I don't think you *get it*. This isn't a game, or a problem to solve. You're in the fight of your life yet you're too damn stubborn and self-willed and judgemental to see it. You're constantly trying to game us, instead of focusing on getting better.' He sighed. 'It's going to take a lot more than a few weeks to break all that down.' He then leaned in and whispered, 'You know I can't recommend you go back to medical school after this. Not in this shape. If something doesn't change soon, you'll never be able to go back at all.'

More tears of self-pity welled and slithered down my cheeks. I nodded. I knew what was coming next. It was something I had wanted to avoid the moment I had arrived and first heard about it, but now my fate was sealed. And there was nothing I could do about it. Refusing would have meant abandoning my dream of becoming a doctor.

I was being transferred to a place called Tabankulu for 'extended primary care'.

Tabankulu was in Kommetjie, a secluded suburb on the outskirts of Cape Town. It had once operated as a farm, with the generous plot of land dominated by a large house for the farmer and his family, speckled with lots of smaller quarters for the workers. There were chicken coops with excitable birds flapping and cooing, and wide-open spaces where fields had either given way to haphazardly mown lawns or been left for the local vegetation to reclaim. In the distance, the peaceful Atlantic was visible, separated by large swathes of fynbos.

The main house had recently been renovated, with a counselling area built as a second floor. Unlike the primary rehab, which oozed sterility and felt like a hospital, Tabankulu had a rustic, slightly shabby feel to it. The carpets were worn in parts, dust motes glided in the shafts of sunlight that poured through the large windows, and the scattered pieces of furniture were dulled and cracked, yet still sturdy, as if to highlight that they had accommodated hundreds of patients over the years and would accommodate many hundreds more.

There was another large whiteboard in the counselling area, with the names of the patients, together with the number of weeks they had been there. Next to Alastair was a '0'. Scanning down the list, I was startled to see some names with an '8', '12' or even '16' next to their name. This was clearly going to be a significantly longer haul than I had originally anticipated.

Later that evening, I met the head of Tabankulu. A slightly overweight man, he had an aura of profound seriousness about him. He gazed at me with the weary look of someone who was tired of my shit even though I hadn't told him anything yet. His thinning hair and deep-set wrinkles suggested he was older than the initial impression made by his youngish-looking face. His eyes were completely neutral, indicating neither happiness nor sadness, interest nor disinterest, at my presence.

After introducing himself as Jim, he got straight to the point. His soft voice sounded exhausted (all the good counsellors sounded exhausted), as if the low volume it operated at was all he could muster.

'What're you hoping to get out of your time here with us, Alastair?' he asked.

'Well, obviously I'd like to get sober. And I'm sick and tired of being sick and tired ...' I glanced up to see if that well-worn AA phrase would impress him, but not a single muscle on his face had moved. Slightly disquieted, I continued, '... and, really, I just want my life back, you know? And I want to get back into medical school.'

'Was your life fun and meaningful?'

'Excuse me?'

Once again, his face was like stone.

'Your life before you got here. You want it back, but was it making you happy?'

I simply stared at him.

'I guess what I'm trying to say is ... was your life worth returning to? Because it seems to me that you're living in a fantasy land. Your girlfriend couldn't wait to break up with you and now never wants to see you again. Not only did your friends not want to live with you, but they also no longer wished to even *hang out* with you. And you've found yourself here, where no one wants to be. It seems to me like your life really wasn't that great.' He paused.

'Also, I would probably forget about medical school if I were you.' He slowly looked me up and down. 'You'll never be a doctor. Find something else to do.'

PART 2: THE HISTORY

I was too shocked to even know how to respond. No one had ever told me that before. Being a doctor was all I had ever wanted to be, and here someone was telling me straight that I simply wasn't cut out for it. Once my brain had processed what he said, a red mist slowly descended over my eyes. Before I could splutter a response, he walked away, calling over his shoulder, 'Welcome to Tabankulu, your last chance.'

That first night was one of the loneliest of my life. I was put into a two-man room with a sullen Welshman who grunted when I introduced myself, and barely made eye contact. The only enthusiasm he seemed to show was during the ravenous inhalations of the cigarettes that he chain-smoked at all hours. For the first night since my relapse I had not been given a sleeping tablet, and anti-depression medication had been started on the advice of the psychiatrist at the primary rehab. I was put onto a hefty dose and the insomnia (which was described as a common side effect) seeped into my consciousness like a high-pitched ring in my head that wouldn't stop. The wind sped over the icy Atlantic and swept through the grounds of the rehab unimpeded. Our room was constructed of corrugated iron, which seemed to bleed away whatever warmth I managed to establish under my blankets. My mind raced from thought to thought, shifting between intense anger at those who had sent me to this hellhole, and self-pity at the thought of being stuck here for weeks on end. When I eventually nodded off, I was woken by the squeaking of the bunk bed as my roommate settled in above me, followed by his groans as he masturbated unselfconsciously. When I eventually fell back asleep, a wan light was peeking through the windows and the roosters were beginning their morning crows.

In many ways Tabankulu was like a repeat of the primary rehab, except played at a much slower speed. We still had to get up every morning at 6am to be ready for the morning Serenity Prayer at 6:45am. We still had P&D groups every day and individual counselling sessions a few times a week, but these were far less intense than they had been in primary care. There was a languid gentleness to activities and everyone seemed to be in less of a rush to get through everything. Afternoons were spent on physical activities around the farm. Although I initially approached these with hesitation, after weeks spent sitting around drinking bad coffee and smoking cigarettes, it felt good to get my hands dirty and my lungs full of fresh air.

Much like my roommate, the people at Tabankulu were nothing like me and this irritated me immensely. They were nice enough people, but they were much heavier drinkers and drug users than I was. Their stories were so much worse than mine.

My mum came to visit me on my third weekend there.

'Al, how are you feeling?'

'Fine, Mum. I just miss home, you know? This is a weird place.'

'Your brother and sister send their love. And Janey McKenzie asked me to tell you that she still remembers when you were five and in nursery school. She remembers that time you cut your eyebrow when the jungle gym fell on top of you and a bunch of other kids. She said you didn't make a single sound until you had made sure everyone else was safe. She says she has never met a braver boy.'

I smiled, remembering my nursery-school teacher, Janey, and how she used to care for me and make me feel safe.

'Your counsellors tell me that they're struggling to get through to you. They think you're holding back. Why is that, my darling?' Her tone was kind and solicitous rather than accusatory. I felt my cheeks starting to burn. I hated being asked these questions by my mum; it brought up all the shame and regret I struggled to keep

PART 2: THE HISTORY

beneath the surface.

'I don't know, Mum. I'm doing my best.' I stared at the floor. I could feel tears welling up.

'Would you like a cup of tea, ma'am?' Mike, my surly roommate, helpfully stepped in. 'By the way, I'm Mike,' he said, in his thick Welsh accent.

'Oh yes. Thank you, Mike.'

Once she had the steaming mug in her hands, and Mike had left, she remarked, 'He seems like a nice young man. What's he doing in here?'

'Oh, Mum, Mike is a crack cocaine user.' I could see the shock on her face and I realised this was an opportunity to direct the spotlight away from me and my shame.

'Yeah,' I went on, remembering what he had said in a recent P&D group, 'he stole a thousand quid from his pregnant girlfriend and went on a massive bender. When that ran out, he sold all their furniture. He even sold the baby books she'd bought and their spot in the antenatal classes his girlfriend had signed them up for. He tried to sell their puppy, but eventually his girlfriend left with it five minutes before a buyer arrived.'

I could tell my mum was taken aback. She was trying to reconcile the polite man who had kindly offered her tea with the story I had told her of someone willing to compromise their future baby's health for another high. I sensed her curiosity had shifted away from me and I decided to press the advantage. I also realised that by telling her how much worse everyone else was, she'd see that keeping me here was all some sort of unexplained cosmic injustice. It played into the notion that, despite it all, I did not belong with these people. I decided to scan the room, and settled on Dirk, a middle-aged guy from Amsterdam.

'See him?' Dirk was playing chess with Gertrude, one of the

volunteers who kept an eye on us over the weekends. His thinning hair was combed over an enlarging bald spot and his lips were pursed in concentration as he pondered his next move.

'What about him?' she said.

'Used to be a respected architect. Hurt his back and had an operation. His surgeon gave him Dilaudid and before he knew it, he was addicted to painkillers.'

'Oh my god. Poor man. That's awful.'

Dirk had found an opening on the board and moved one of his pawns. But then his frown deepened, and he gingerly moved it back. His fingers returned to his temples, which he massaged thoughtfully.

'Yeah,' I decided to carry on unprompted, 'he was so high, he passed out driving his daughters home from school. Smashed into a tree. Everyone was fine but his wife had had enough and left with the kids. He carried on using for another two years.'

This continued for the next thirty minutes. I'd identify someone and explain the shocking or terrible things they had done. There was a thrill to it; the same feeling you get when sharing a particularly juicy piece of gossip or revealing a dirty secret. Words tumbled out of me in a way they never did during the group sessions. The more shocked my mum became, the more I felt emboldened to continue. Suddenly, the drab days spent listening to imploding lives became noteworthy. But more importantly, my words identified me as a reporter, not as a participant. Through this distinction, I was attempting to distance myself from the other patients in my mother's eyes. By the time visiting hours were over, I felt cleansed, like I had emerged from confession.

'Alastair, do you have anything you want to tell us?' Jim's voice was hard, different to the anodyne tone he had adopted when he had first welcomed me to Tabankulu. The eyes of the group were on me and I could feel I was walking into a trap. I swallowed and felt sweat prick on my neck and back.

'Uh ... about what?'

'About what you told your mother yesterday.'

'What do you mean?'

Jim sighed and leaned forward. 'The things we discuss in group are totally confidential. They're so confidential we read a statement to that effect before each one. People here need to know that they are in a safe space and that what they share will be respected. It's an environment built on trust. Yesterday, you violated that trust.' He paused, letting the words settle on me like a net.

'Gertrude overheard just about everything you said. Unlike you, she actually listens.'

Rivulets of sweat were running down my back and from under my arms. A suffocating darkness closed in around me. I felt the eyes of all the other patients boring through my skin. I stared at the floor and kneaded my knuckles over and over.

'How does the group feel about this?' he asked.

'Seriously, fuck you, man. My life isn't a joke and my addiction isn't either. Who the fuck are you to think you can look down on us?' said one guy.

'What a fucking prick you are,' said another.

'Some of us are trying to get better, you know. If you don't want to, you don't have to. But the least you can do is shut up about it.'

The waves of shame rolled over me. Everyone hated me. How was I going to survive many more weeks of this?

Jim calmed the group down. When he next spoke, his voice remained diamond-hard.

'The thing is ... this is a serious violation of our rules. I have spoken with the other counsellors and we considered kicking you out, but there's nowhere else for you to go. We're at the end of the line here. If we do kick you out, you would not complete the programme. Your medical school won't take you back without a fulsome endorsement from us and let me tell you, at this rate, that simply isn't going to happen.

'Alastair, you really need to think about what you're even doing here. It's clear that weeks of rehab haven't got through that layer you've constructed around yourself. Time is running out. And now this. Does anyone have anything else to add?'

'I do.' It was Mike, who'd been so kind to my mum and who I'd repaid with betrayal.

'Mate, when I first heard what you'd done, how you'd broken your promise to us for a few laughs, I wanted to punch your fucking lights out. But the more I thought about it, the more I just felt sorry for you. You're, like, the dumbest smart person I've ever met. Help is literally being offered to you on a platter and still you refuse to take it. You have friends and colleagues and family all cheering for you. You have this amazing life to live. And still you fuck around. I've come to terms with the things I did. Have you? I actually *want* to get better. Do you?'

As punishment, I was excluded from all group activities for one week. I had to eat alone and wasn't allowed any visitors. While everyone enjoyed the weekend leisure activities (like braaiing or watching a movie), I had to cut logs for the fire, clean out the chicken coops and wash all the dishes and cooking equipment. Even when I could interact with others, I simply received glares and a palpable silence when I tried to initiate conversation.

The hard labour wasn't a problem, but the loneliness was physically choking and reminded me of lying in my bed, alone, drunk and staring at my phone.

Five days into my punishment, while chopping wood, it started

PART 2: THE HISTORY

to rain. It was the middle of winter and I had not brought any gloves with me. My hands were so cold that after chopping a few logs, releasing the axe became almost impossible as my fingers were frozen in position. I glanced inside the main house and saw the other patients playing charades, drinking bad coffee and laughing together. Water dripped off my eyebrows into my eyes and my nose had started to run. Each heave of the axe seemed to miss its target or get stuck in a soft part of the wood, requiring painful wriggling to extricate it.

I looked up and saw Jim walking towards me and I thought he was coming to tell me to get inside, but he was simply dropping off more logs to be cut.

'Tired of being alone?' The logs crashed down next to me. Whatever hopes I had of going inside anytime soon were dashed; the counsellors had made it clear I could only go in when all the wood had been chopped.

I heaved the axe up and brought it down as hard as I could, savouring the jolt that shot through my arms.

'You think no one will ever understand your shame, Alastair. You think if people saw who you really are and what you've done, they would reject you. So you project an image – the cocky, controlled, smart medical student. The guy who can think his way out of anything. Except now there's something you can't reason against, or bargain with, or outwit, or bring to heel with clever wordplay. You have a *disease*. It's bigger than you. It's consuming you. All your coping mechanisms have brought you here. Being cold, chopping wood in the rain, your future wrecked, your life going nowhere slowly. An ex-girlfriend you're still in love with but to whom you are so unrecognisable she nearly called the cops out of fear, a medical-school itching – and I mean *itching* – to expel you. And now, even in here, surrounded by people trying to help you get better, you insist on staying in your dark hole.'

The axe came down again, neatly splitting a log into two.

'What do you want me to do?'

'Time to stop getting your arse kicked. Time to stop fighting.'

'But ... *how*, Jim? I can't stand it here. Look at what you're making me do.'

'Oh for Christ's sake, Alastair. This is hardly a Russian gulag. You have three meals a day and a warm bed. You're not even a prisoner. You could literally walk out the front gate right now and no one would stop you. Yet still you complain and whine. At the first sign of suffering, you act like you're bloody Solzhenitsyn.'

Another axe blow found its mark. I wiped my brow, savouring the slickness of the icy rain and the warm sweat.

'This is too big for you. It's not your fault you have this disease, but you are responsible for your recovery. But you'll need to use that brain of yours to stop fighting.'

'But how, Jim? Seriously, man. How do you stop fighting?'

He gave me one final glance as he strolled away. Then he paused, turned around again, and said softly, 'Have you considered asking for help?'

That evening, after warming my bleeding and blistered hands, I decided to call my ex-girlfriend. There was a public phone which I picked up and gingerly tapped the keys with my aching fingers. Her number was burned into my brain and almost seemed to dial itself. After a few rings, I heard a familiar 'Hello?'

For a moment, I was completely speechless. I had missed hearing the calming timbre of her voice. The way it inflected down rather than up, making it seem like she was expecting your call.

'Hey. It's Al.' There was a long pause and an audible exhalation.

'Why are you calling me?'

PART 2: THE HISTORY

'Because I miss you. I miss you so much. I really just need ...'

'Alastair. You need to stop.' The finality cut through like a blade. 'You're stuck. But I'm not the one to help you. I can't. With Dad's death ...' she began to sob, '... I just can't. Why won't you leave me alone? Please just leave me alone—'

'But you never visit ...'

'I *did* visit! Or were you too drunk to remember?'

'That was because the counsellors made you come. Not because you wanted to.'

'You think ... you think I did that for anyone other than *you*? I was trying to help you! Did you consider, for a single moment, the toll that took on me?'

'Why won't you come again?'

'Because now I don't *want* to visit you. It hurts too much. Can't you *see*?' She sobbed again before regaining her composure. My heart was hammering in my chest and my mouth was dry.

'I need to tell you something,' she finally murmured. 'I'm seeing someone.'

'What? I mean ... what does that mean?' My thoughts crossed and smudged each other out. I couldn't think straight.

'He's really good to me. He's kind. I know this will upset you, but you were going to hear about it sooner or later. I thought it would be the kindest coming from me. I hope you understand.'

'Do I know him?' I almost convulsed over the words.

'No. And please – please! – don't cause a scene like you did last time. Give me this. Give me this peace. I beg you.' A male voice I didn't recognise was discernible in the background.

'Is that him?' I asked.

'I have to go. Please don't call again.' The line went dead. It felt like an eternity before I was able to return the phone to its cradle.

I felt numb. Initially, I was too shocked to do anything. Mike must have seen my face because he came over, put a hand on my shoulder and asked if I was okay. That did it. Like a dam bursting its walls, the tears poured forth. It was as if his kind gesture was the final crack of the pickaxe that shattered the ice. I wept until it felt like I had no tears left. When I eventually stopped, it felt like I had excavated below sadness and hit upon blank nothingness. I was suddenly overwhelmingly tired. Every muscle in my body ached, yet when I went to bed, I couldn't sleep. The thoughts of the past few weeks in rehab, the shame of the addiction, the misery of that final call to my ex ... I was nowhere near being in a place of rest. Eventually, in sheer desperation, I followed Jim's advice and did something I hadn't done since I was a teenager: I asked a higher power for help.

I was not religious at that time, and I'm not religious now, but at that point I simply didn't have any other options. I closed my eyes and I prayed. I didn't care who was listening, but it was time to try something different, and I was too tired and drained to think of anything else.

I breathed deeply and tried to still my mind. I savoured how my lungs felt when they filled with air. I noted the dried patches of salt where tears had rolled down my cheeks. I felt the hammering in my chest and how, almost imperceptibly, it began to slow to a more normal rate. The darkness behind my eyes lightened very gradually, becoming a deep and soothing blue. I gulped and my thoughts began racing. The blue began to fade and something inside me told me that to keep it, I needed to speak. Aloud. So I did.

I got out of bed, knelt beside it and began murmuring softly.

I admitted that my life was a mess. It was a mess because I couldn't stop drinking. But it was more than that. It was a mess because everything was about me. It was a mess because I was incapable of being honest about my feelings to anyone, least of all myself. It was a mess because I thought I had the ability to get myself out of this, when all the evidence showed that my own attempts were simply digging myself deeper. It was a mess because I still believed I could find my own way through without any help.

Please help me. Please.

I realised that asking to be suddenly healed was simply an extension of my selfishness again, so I asked to be shown what to do and to be assisted in finding the courage to do it. I said I would stop fighting and do whatever the counsellors asked of me. I stated that I would be as honest as possible, even if the shame was overwhelming.

I don't know if anyone was listening. Perhaps it doesn't matter. But I do know that after I finished, the deep, soothing blue stayed with me until I fell asleep. I felt peace for the first time in a very long time. A calmness descended over me and the sadness was lifted. When I awoke, nothing was different, but suddenly everything was. The words came unbidden: 'God, grant me the serenity to accept the things I cannot change, the courage to change the things I can, and the wisdom to know the difference.'

The next day in the group session, I took a leap. I told everyone how, despite having no prior intention of doing so, I had got drunk at my cousin's wedding a year before. I started drinking gin before we even left for the church, made a fool of myself at the table and embarrassed my family by hitting the dance floor before the bride and groom had finished their first dance, taking the attention away from them on their special night. Shortly thereafter, I had vomited on myself, passed out in the garden, and had to be supported home. I woke the next day with a terrible headache and very little memory of what had happened. Not terrible in the grand scheme of things, but I knew I had caused my family great shame and made a dreadful fool of myself.

When I was done, I took a deep breath.

Jim looked at me. 'Do you see how alcohol robs you of your agency? How you had no intention of passing out in a cold garden while everyone else was having fun? But once you started, you were simply unable to moderate your intake?'

I nodded.

'How does telling us that make you feel?'

I knew what I was supposed to say. I knew the answer the group was expecting to hear was shame. Shame at my behaviour. Remorse. A desire to change. But that wasn't the predominant emotion raging in my chest, so I paused. Then I stopped thinking and spoke without thinking too much about it.

'I'm angry. I'm so fucking angry I could choke. Why has this happened to me? Why am I here? Why can I not drink again? You people expect me to abstain for ... what? ... ever? How? A kid in his twenties just drinking Coke while everyone else is having fun? I'll *never* fit in. I should never have let this happen. I should have been stronger. Why am I so fucking *weak*?'

I stopped suddenly. Everyone was looking at me, but something was different. Mike looked at me. 'I think that's one of the first truly honest things you've shared with us. For the first time, I believe the words coming out of your mouth.'

That night, sleep did not come. There was an uncomfortable pressure in my chest. I felt like a spider painfully shedding its skin. Everything was itchy and uncomfortable.

I replayed the day in my head, feeling alternately relieved and embarrassed. I was worried that I had deviated from the expected script and that it would be used to keep me back. I kept shifting and turning.

Eventually, the light came on. My roommate had had enough.

'Can't sleep, yeah?' he said in a thick Welsh lilt. 'Like your body is exhausted but your head is swimmin' a million miles per hour? Try this.'

'What is it?'

'Never mind. It might help. Or it might make you mental.' He grinned, exposing teeth stained by nicotine. He thrust a blank CD into my hand. I hesitantly took out my Discman and popped it in. I put my headphones on and closed my eyes.

It started peacefully enough. A lone acoustic guitar playing lilting chords that thrummed pleasantly in my ears. It wasn't revolutionary stuff, and I could imagine trying to meditate to it, but it was relaxing. I settled down and crossed my arms over each other, cradling my elbows.

The acoustic guitar switched effortlessly to electric, but remained restrained and gentle, with basic melodic changes and pleasing harmonic shifts. My mind started wandering again, with a million thoughts vying for my attention. I was about to shift my focus back to my anxieties when it happened.

I initially thought something was wrong with my headphones. An utterly thunderous wall of sound suddenly crashed into my ears. My brain retaliated by rejecting what it was hearing. Everything was wrong. Drums were blasting at a speed that felt impossibly fast. Guitars were so loud and distorted that I could barely make them out. When riffs did emerge, they were so angular and prickly that it felt like a cactus was being rubbed against my ear drums. Then an unearthly shriek pierced the cacophony, sounding only peripherally human, like a creature drowning in boiling water. Or a demon dredged from a sewer. It was frankly mesmerising in its ugliness. The addition of synthesisers and choral voices only added to the confusion I was hearing. It sounded as if it had been recorded in someone's basement on a cassette deck.

I was a fan of rock, including some of the harder stuff, but this was on a whole different level. I wasn't sure it could be called music. I took my headphones off.

'Mate. This is ... just not my thing. Sorry.'

My roommate was looking at me with a glint in his eye. 'Stop being a wimp and just listen to the whole song. Just one song.' I could feel that this was some kind of test. And I didn't know how long I'd have to share a room with him, so I put the headphones back on and gritted my teeth as the clanging fury enveloped me. The track did not improve over its five-minute runtime, but it didn't become any worse either. By the end, I could even make out the hint of a melody or two. When it concluded, I popped the Discman and handed the CD back to him.

'Emperor,' he said, followed by 'Black metal,' as if that would mean anything to me or explain what I had just heard. He pressed again. 'What do you think?'

'I've never heard of "Emperor",' I conceded. 'Or "black metal". I didn't really know there were different types of metal. To be honest, I'm more an indie-rock kinda guy. That music is not really my thing. It's just so very ... *loud*. And I don't really like to be screamed at. Sorry.'

'Fair enough. Metal really isn't for everyone. Not everyone can take the journey to hell and back. But I got just one question for ya.'

'Oh yeah? What?'

'What were you worried about while that was going on?'

'Uh ...' I wracked my brain. The clanging had been so all-consuming that I hadn't really been worried about anything. It was like my brain had short-circuited. 'Nothing,' I finally admitted.

He broke into the biggest grin I'd seen from him since I arrived. 'Exactly.'

Over the following weeks, I began to heal. I apologised to everyone

I had betrayed; I shared everything I could during group sessions. With every disclosure, a weight was imperceptibly lifted off me, like a small pebble from a huge mound. I became so desperate to get it all out that during the feedback sessions I was told to dial it back to give others a chance. I shared my shame and my anger and inadequacies without any thought. Like extracting a poison, I wanted it all out.

I joined the afternoon volleyball practice, the morning yoga classes and the evening jogs, relishing the feeling of my dormant muscles moving again.

At night, I was subjected to the yells, screams and blasts of my roommate playing his metal music. My cautious endorsement of that one song had given him the confidence to start playing it through the speaker he kept on his desk. Curiously enough, as time went on, I started to mind less and less when it came on. One of the treatments for children with attention deficit hyperactivity disorder (ADHD) is to give them stimulants. Intuitively, giving something to jack up a hyperactive child seems like a terrible idea, but the stimulant paradoxically focuses their minds, allowing them to concentrate better. For me, the metal music I was listening to acted similarly. Where others found the cacophony stroke-inducing, I found it soothing and focusing, like an all-consuming, protective blanket flung over my smouldering mind, extinguishing the overheated anxieties and fears. I could barely make out a single word among the grunts, growls, yelps and shrieks, but it didn't matter. The words didn't matter. They were simply an abstract expression of emotion I could lose myself in.

Put simply, the vocalists were screaming so that I didn't have to. The music was furious so I didn't have to be. It destroyed things so that I could keep them intact. It was an outlet, one I was appreciating more and more.

I closed my eyes and in the unrelenting maelstrom of fury, in the crashing guitars and thunderous drums, in the dissonance and chaos, I found ... peace.

I came to learn over the following months that while I was not responsible for my alcoholism, I *was* responsible for my recovery. I was drawn to a core group of patients who seemed determine to find sobriety and I stopped hanging out with those just waiting to relapse again.

The anti-depressants I had been prescribed began to kick in, and as the fog of depression started to lift, I discovered I had more energy and enthusiasm to read and write.

I collected first my 30-day and then my 60-day sobriety keyrings from the local NA meetings, which I proudly kept on my person at all times. Whenever I felt the urge to drink, I'd thumb the keyring and silently repeat: 'God, grant me the serenity to accept the things I cannot change, the courage to change the things I can, and the wisdom to know the difference.'

I was invited to share my story as the main speaker in some meetings and I was given more responsibility for managing day-to-day affairs at the rehab. One day Jim approached me, running his hand through his hair, which seemed to thin more every time I saw him.

'I have to say, Alastair, that your transformation has been ... remarkable. There was enormous frustration among the counsellors at your lack of progress in the first five weeks. Yet here you are, ten weeks in, maintaining real sobriety. That's impressive.'

I couldn't resist asking him. It had been on my mind for weeks.

'Still think I could never be a doctor?'

He paused and I could see this was a question that had caught him off guard, but that he nevertheless wanted to answer seriously.

PART 2: THE HISTORY

Weighing every word, as if they were precious gems, he said, 'I've changed my mind. I know you think you *could* be a doctor ...' I could barely hide the smile that was spreading across my lips. '... but I don't think you *should* be a doctor.'

Everything sank. 'It's too stressful,' he continued. 'The long days and nights; the proximity to a variety of tempting drugs; the lack of sleep; the weird eating habits ... these spell disaster for someone in recovery. All it takes is one slip and everything is over. Just one really terrible day. One patient who dies unexpectedly, perhaps due to a mistake you made, and you're back to square one. Every single day you are one relapse from ending your career. Forever. I just don't think it's worth it.'

'But it's the only thing I've ever wanted to do.'

'You're a talented guy. You're smart. There are lots of roads to happiness. You can find something else. I'm just not sure you're strong enough for what's coming.' He gave me a meaningful look that spoke of personal experience.

'Please, Jim. Please. I can't go back to medical school without your report telling them you're satisfied with my recovery.'

'So all of this ... is just to go back? You'll need a stronger reason than that to stay sober.'

'It's not. You know it's not. I'm sober because I want to be sober. But I also want to pursue my dream. Please, Jim. Please write that report.'

'And what if I said that we want you to stay a bit longer?'

I gulped. In my head, I was ten days shy of three months at Tabankulu. This was usually as long as most people stayed unless there were extenuating circumstances.

'How much longer?'

'Four weeks.'

I didn't hesitate. 'Done.'

'Just like that?'

'Just like that.'

He strolled away, whistling to himself and muttering, 'This place is always so full of surprises ...'

After three and a half months at Tabankulu, I was finally ready to leave and try secondary rehab again. Except this time, I had no intention of drinking. I would be able to reconnect with my life and start doing normal things again.

In December that year, I was informed that, barring any relapses, I would be able to start medical school the following January, but I would have to repeat fourth year.

It was time to start life again.

Chapter 11
SIPHO AND THE BEETROOT

RESTARTING FOURTH YEAR OF MEDICAL SCHOOL WAS A CONFLICTING EXPERIENCE. On the one hand I was grateful to be back; my medical career had hung in the balance for so long that it was a huge relief to return. On the other, I felt lonely and exposed. All my friends were in the year above me, and I was starting over with a group of people I barely knew, but who were all comfortable and familiar with each other after three gruelling pre-clinical years. In addition, I knew that they were all aware why I was joining them. The wounds of recovery were fresh and I was uncomfortable exposing them. I was finding my way and I still felt incredibly raw and sensitive, especially outside my circle of recovery.

To some extent, while I had been in rehab, I had been sheltered from all things non-recovery. The focus on myself was so intense, and my life so completely geared towards making it through another day sober, that it was easy to forget that outside the walls of rehab, the world had carried on as usual for everyone else. Now I felt naked. To the other people in the room I wasn't the guy who had clawed his way to six months of sobriety; I was simply Alastair, the dude who drank too much, found himself in rehab, and was held back a year.

During registration I felt like I was under a white-hot spotlight. Every smirk, every glance, every giggle seemed magnified. My new classmates were polite and friendly, but I could see the curiosity in their eyes. I stood out for all the wrong reasons. As someone who craved respect, this was deeply humbling. I tried to convince myself that it didn't matter what other people thought of me. This provided some mild relief, but I could still feel my heart racing.

Returning to med school had come with caveats: I had to stay sober; I had to see a psychiatrist every three months; I had to continue attending AA/NA meetings and support groups. It was made abundantly clear to me that I was skating on extremely thin ice; the committee had been split about whether to allow me back at all. Only the glowing reports from my counsellors (Jim, in particular) had swayed them. One false move, however, and I would be permanently expelled.

My life was very different to how it had been the previous year. Most evenings consisted of going to AA or NA meetings. I had found myself a sponsor to help me work through the Twelve-Step Program and I was working on the infamous Step 4 ('We made a thorough and searching inventory of ourselves'). This involved a relentlessly uncompromising introspection and documentation of my character. Like lifting a rock in a garden, not everything that was exposed was pleasant, and many of the truths about my defects were plain and inescapable. There's a reason Step 4 has such a fearsome reputation in recovery circles.

I was living with a guy I had met at secondary care and spent most of my time with him and other recovery buddies.

Fourth year of medical school was a clinical year at UCT. Most of the week was spent in hospitals, shadowing doctors and seeing patients. I had started doing this the previous year but going back felt completely different. When you've been a patient, even a psychiatric one, for any period of time, you gain a unique perspective on what it's like to be on the other side of the stethoscope. The fear, the uncertainty, the loneliness. But you also pick up the little things. The doctor whose eyes keep darting to the door is a doctor who has stopped listening and is in a hurry to leave. The doctor who tries to bend your answers into a preconceived diagnosis is not someone willing to be flexible in the face of conflicting information. The doctor who isn't interested in learning the pronunciation of your name is not particularly interested in the nuances of your pain. The doctor who sizes you up in one look and makes up his mind before you even open your mouth is the doctor you can't trust opening yourself up to. And the doctor who refers to you by your diagnosis ('The knee in bed 12,' 'The alcoholic in room 4') has stopped seeing you as a person and thinks of you as a problem to be solved.

When admitting and examining (what we referred to as 'clerking') patients, I sometimes found their suffering overwhelming. Having been in the dark pit of despair myself, revisiting that pit in others was a journey I was simply not yet fully equipped to undertake. So, initially, I hid behind the refuge of academics.

If patients were puzzles to be solved rather than humans in pain, I could shield myself from my own uncomfortable emotions. It helped that many of the senior clinicians around me seemed to feel the same way. When doing tutorials or teaching, these doctors were perfectly professional and polite. They sought patient permission before examining them in front of students, and the patients seemed satisfied with the care they were receiving. But it became clear early on that we were all predominantly focused on the patients' pathologies. We spent hours discussing unusual clinical findings, differential diagnoses and the latest treatment modalities. We spent little time on the patients' hopes and fears, their anxieties, the gnawing voice inside them wondering who would look after their pets if they suddenly died.

During one ward round, I presented Mr Peterson, who was extremely close to his dog, a Labrador named Chuck. I mentioned to the consultant that the patient wasn't sleeping at night because he was worried that Chuck was lonely in his absence. There was an awkward silence before I heard some coughing and stifled laughter. The consultant grinned. 'Unless you think ... what was his name again ... Chuck? Unless you think Chuck has any meaningful effect on Mr Peterson's inflammatory bowel disease, we can probably leave that stuff to the social workers.' He couldn't have been more wrong. Chuck the Labrador played a pivotal role during the flare-up. While the anxiety persisted, Mr Peterson's illness proved refractory to everything we tried. In desperation, I contacted his trusted neighbour who agreed to look after Chuck, take him in, and make sure he was fed and loved. I relayed this to Mr Peterson and instantly I could see the anxiety flow out of him like pus being drained from an abscess. His inflammation subsequently settled. The consultant took the credit because of the introduction of a fancy new medication, and maybe that did the trick, but I now make sure to ask every patient the names of their pets and who's looking after them.

Surrounded by suffering, I sometimes wondered whether the job description was simply too much. If humans are fundamentally ill-equipped to spend so much time around so much pain and illness. I asked a very senior colleague who had practised for fifty years, always with a smile on his face, how he did it. How had he managed to stay immune to the darkness around him, day in and day out?

'Alastair, every morning I wake up with an emotional biscuit jar and that determines how many emotional biscuits I'm willing to expend on that day.'

He saw my perplexed expression and laughed. 'Yeah, it's a bit trite, but hear me out. On any given day, I wake up with a certain number of biscuits in my jar. Depending on how tired I am, how disruptive the kids were at dinner time, if I had a fight with my wife, how stressful work has been ... these all determine how many biscuits I have. Now, as the day goes on, I expend my biscuits on my patients. But here's the thing. When the jar is empty, then it's *empty*. I don't give out biscuits I don't have. Too many doctors do. It's why they burned out and I didn't.'

'How do you know when you've got to the bottom of the jar?' I asked.

'Oh man! You know! You feel it deep in here.' He pointed to his bulging abdomen. 'It's when that *tiredness* sets in, you know? That fatigue that you feel deep in your bloody bones.'

'But what happens if, like, it's only lunch time and your jar is empty, but you still have an afternoon's worth of patients to see?'

'Then you stay cool and professional and you do your best to sort them out, but you don't invest any personal emotional energy. They cry? You give them a tissue. They tell you about their family troubles? You listen quietly. But you don't invest. See? Don't overdo it with those biscuits and you'll be okay.' He happened to be holding a chocolate-chip biscuit in his hand at that very moment. He looked at it as if it was some cosmic proof of his point, took a generous bite and cheerfully shuffled off.

I often think about that conversation. Was it a simple metaphor hiding a deeper truth? Or an over-simplified justification for being a bit of an ass sometimes? It was a truism that too many doctors were so tired that they began their days with very little emotional energy. Between brutal training, long hours, debt, stress, paperwork and the emotional suffering they were around every day, there was often not much left to give. But it also struck me that this may have been a cop-out – a pithy excuse the physician told himself when he simply couldn't be bothered to make the effort to care. All these years later, I believe the answer may lie somewhere in the middle.

I could see the crown of the slimy, slightly bloody head.

'Support the perineum!'

I snapped out of my trance and put my hand just beneath the woman's vulva, trying to support it.

'Don't tickle it, young man, that's her husband's job! Support!' The nurse was commanding and no-nonsense in her tone, but not unkind. We had been waiting for this moment for the past forty-five minutes. Ms February was well into the second stage of labour, and for the first time I could see the baby I was supposed to be delivering. I gulped. Obstetrics and gynaecology was my first block of the year. Like all the others to come, it was three months long. During that time, I was expected to observe at least five deliveries and personally deliver fifteen babies. Part of it was spent in Mitchells Plain, a small offshoot of Cape Town where, decades before, the apartheid government had forcibly relocated hundreds of so-called 'coloured' families from Cape Town in an effort to separate the races. Unlike the leafy suburbs of Newlands, Mitchells Plain was flat, windy and sandy. Years later, the scars of apartheid still lingered in the form of poverty, drug abuse and gangsterism. Nevertheless, we had to learn that there was more to obstetrics than delivering babies in the hushed corridors of tertiary hospitals like Groote Schuur and part of our rotation was in more peripheral maternity obstetric units (MOUs). Although I never felt unsafe, I only had to look beyond the property fence to see the often-violent world of the Cape Flats.

The world of the pre-clinical years, epitomised by studying dry textbooks in the air-conditioned campus library, seemed a million miles away.

I had watched videos on delivering babies during student orientation. I had read the textbooks and seen the diagrams. I knew the theory of how a woman's body miraculously managed to get a small human through a small opening in the pelvis, and an even smaller opening in the vagina. It seemed improbable in theory and impossible in reality. I had observed a few deliveries first-hand, but this was different. No textbook prepared me for the odours, the lights and the intimacy of it all. There was no doubt: this was a sacred space. And I was slap-bang in the middle of it.

Ms February let out a shriek and the baby's head millimetred closer to me. I pushed up from the bottom of the perineum.

'Okay, baby's coming. Get ready!' The room stood still. All went quiet. I breathed heavily behind my mask, the weight of what was happening resting uncomfortably on my aching shoulders. This was it. If I got this wrong, this baby would suffer the consequences for the rest of its life. I looked up at Ms February, whose hand was gripping my shoulder so tightly I thought she might dislocate it. Unfortunately, the excitement of the baby's imminent arrival was short-lived. It was a false alarm. The contraction abated and with it the head receded. We were back to where we were a few minutes ago.

Any sense or level of decorum had long since vanished. Ms February's legs were wide open and my head was inches from her vagina. Blood and amniotic fluid stained the sheets around us. She was sweating profusely and continuously jammed her knee into my face with each contraction, after which she would apologise profusely, before another contraction hit. Her boyfriend was pacing nearby, a cigarette tucked behind his ear that he kept reaching for and then mournfully replacing when he realised he couldn't smoke in the room. He knew that stepping outside for a few merciful puffs would bring down such a torrent of cussing and swearing from his girlfriend that he would be made to regret his decision for a very long time.

After another painful contraction, Ms February looked at the midwife standing beside me. 'Sister. I don't think I can.' She was nineteen. This was her first delivery. She had been in labour for nearly twenty-four hours and she was utterly exhausted. The drugs we had put up to expedite the labour didn't seem to be making any difference and the pain medications seemed equally ineffective. 'I don't think I can do this,' she reiterated.

Sister Mpofu was having none of it.

'Hawu! Do you think that baby is going to coming *running* out your vagina? The theatres are full so this baby is not coming out the sunroof. You have to puuuuuuuuush!'

Ms February summoned what little energy she had left and pushed again. Every fibre and ligament in her body tensed. The head inched closer before stopping again. We were at a critical juncture. The baby had been in the second stage of labour (when the cervix is fully dilated to the time of delivery) for too long and was beginning to show signs of distress. We needed to get this baby out.

'In soos 'n piesang, uit soos 'n pynappel. Episiotomy time.' Sister Mpofu handed me what looked like the largest, scariest set of scissors I had ever seen. 'Make the cut to make more room for the baby.'

I gulped again. I knew, in theory, what I should be doing, but once the scissors were in my hand, it was a different experience altogether.

'Shouldn't the doctor be doing this?' I whispered to Sister Mpofu, while trying to look calm for Ms February's benefit.

'He's in theatre doing a caesarean section, Alastair. The intern is managing a post-partum haemorrhage in room 4. You're it.' She saw the panicked look on my face. 'Don't worry. I'll help you.'

Time seemed to go very slowly at that point and then very quickly. While I had been gathering myself, Sister Mpofu had injected the lignocaine into the labia to numb the area for the pain. She directed my hands to the correct spot and told me to be firm, but not too firm. Gentle, but not too gentle. The scissors were sharp and cut the flesh easily. With the extra space, the baby's head seemed to pop out a bit further. It was so close. Ms February let out a high-pitched howl with the next contraction.

Sister Mpofu looked at her patient. Her features briefly softened.

'Sisi. I know you're tired. But baby needs to come. All this screaming is wasting energy. That baby is not coming out of the mouth. Focus. And puuuuuuuuuuuush!'

This time it was different. Ms February pulled every ounce of energy she had left from a well deep within her. Her forehead crinkled, but other than a short grunt, she made no further sound. Every ounce of energy was focused on that final effort. The baby's crown advanced further and further and suddenly … it popped out. I supported the head as it gently turned.

'Now ease out the shoulder,' instructed Sister Mpofu. I didn't seem to do much when the top shoulder appeared and, with a gush, the entire baby emerged. It was blue and covered in creamy vernix and blood. But it was silent. Sister Mpofu was cutting the umbilical cord, but all eyes were on me. The only sound in the room was the gentle beeping of the saturation monitor, but my ears were filled with white noise. I don't think I'd ever heard such a deafening silence.

'Hawu, don't just stand there! Help it!'

The resus bay was a few feet away. I swaddled the baby and placed it on the tray. Ms February's boyfriend was standing next to me.

'What's wrong? Do we need a doctor? We should get a real doctor.'

'Just give me a sec,' I grunted. I vigorously rubbed the baby to warm it. I then dried it and scooped some fluid out of its mouth. There was a brief cough, and then, like an engine sputtering to life, a low whine emerged from the little bundle in front of me. The whine soon blossomed into a furious howl and the whole room seemed to exhale. The tension in the room suddenly shifted to joy.

'Is it a boy or girl?' asked Ms February.

I realised that in all the chaos I had forgotten to check.

'A girl.'

Ms February started sobbing. Her boyfriend followed suit and once again reached for, and then abandoned, his cigarette. I swaddled the baby and took her to her exhausted mother and placed her on her chest.

'Congratulations,' I whispered.

'I'll deliver the placenta and do the suturing. You look like you need to sit down,' Sister Mpofu said to me.

I raced to the students' office and put my head between my hands, which were shaking uncontrollably. It was hard to tell what was louder: the sobs of relief or the gasps for air that wouldn't seem to enter my lungs. I was glad that no one was around to see the tears streaming down my cheeks.

If my obstetrics and gynaecology block was about life, then the internal medicine block that followed was about grappling with death. While it is a constant presence in hospitals, and something doctors learn to make an uneasy truce with, this was different. We were not holding it at bay. Instead, death was invasive and corrosive. It seeped through the walls and under the doors. It stole through the night without mercy. It wasn't swift and sure, but slow and

PART 2: THE HISTORY

excruciating. It lingered on bed linen. It was on everyone's lips but was hardly ever said out loud. An epidemic of shame and suffering that we were powerless to stop. HIV.

HIV put healthcare workers in an impossible situation. In the early 2000s, President Thabo Mbeki had decided that HIV did not cause AIDS ('How can a virus cause a syndrome?' he had famously said, pontificating with a pipe firmly clenched in his lips) and that the problem had been blown completely out of proportion. A quick internet search over his morning coffee had shown him that HIV was *not* among the leading causes of death in South Africa at the time. Why, he wondered, were we all fretting about it so much? Logical explanations from experts that, like an engine leaking fuel, HIV depleted the immune system until something else administered the *coup de grâce*, which confounded official statistics, fell on deaf ears. Mbeki ruled the majority African National Congress (ANC) party with an iron fist and those around him either sycophantically agreed or were too afraid to voice their opposition. Indeed, to prove his point, Mbeki held a conference in Durban in 2000 where he invited known HIV deniers and cranks to speak, all of whom confirmed his biases. AIDS was caused by poverty and malnutrition, not HIV, they claimed. HIV itself was, at most, an innocent bystander and by throwing toxic drugs at it we were making it worse. What South Africans needed, these pseudo-experts pronounced, were 'African solutions to African problems'.

The pan-Africanist in Mbeki was delighted. South Africa would forge its own path, rejecting the attempts by the West to recolonise it through economic dependence on drugs it didn't need. As a result, patients with HIV in South Africa were not eligible to receive antiretroviral therapy, which was available elsewhere in the world. Dr Manto Tshabalala-Msimang, South Africa's then minister of health, enthusiastically promoted an alternative in the form of a concoction of African potato, garlic, lemon and beetroot, invoking a return to traditional values and therapies. When shocked scientists pointed out that the African potato could be harmful to the liver in the doses recommended by Tshabalala-Msimang, she doubled down, earning herself the nickname, 'Dr Beetroot'.

The results of this ignorance and utter arrogance were predictable and catastrophic. South Africans, mostly black and poor, became sick by the tens of thousands. Young women, in particular, bore the brunt of the epidemic. Hospitals were flooded with people who were slowly and painfully dying; people who we as doctors were powerless to help properly. Even though in 2002 the courts in South Africa ordered the government to provide pregnant women with the drug nevirapine to prevent transmission of the virus to their newborn babies, the government's response was lackadaisical and unfocused. Mbeki continued to claim that the drugs were 'toxic' and resisted a universal roll-out. When he opined that he personally didn't know anyone who had died of HIV, it was a slap in the face for those of us who had watched helplessly as thousands were consumed by the disease.

Most ICUs were so overwhelmed, and the prognosis for these patients so poor, that having HIV or AIDS was regarded as a contraindication for admission. As a result, the care for the dying fell to those of us working in the wards. There is no feeling of despair more profound than watching someone die whose death you know was preventable. There is no anger more visceral than witnessing human misery caused by political ignorance.

The depression and frustration among doctors was palpable and universal. The reactions, however, were varied. Some simply disregarded the government and found alternate ways of sourcing some of the life-saving drugs. They risked their medical licences to do what they thought was right. A doctor I worked with was so determined to reduce mother-to-child transmission that she had a secret stash of antiretrovirals that she would give to HIV-positive mothers in labour, regardless of whether the pharmacy was stocked or not.

Some found themselves burned out by the moral injury they suffered on a daily basis, and retreated behind withering cynicism, doing the best that they could while building a wall between themselves and the tsunami of misery they were confronted with.

Some agreed with Mbeki and felt that providing such powerful and expensive drugs to so many poor people was a fool's errand, especially in a developing country like South Africa. How on earth could we expect poor and uneducated folk to be compliant with such complicated medications? they mused. Best to wait it out, not bankrupt ourselves fighting the inevitable, and pick up the pieces afterwards.

Some used it as an avenue to express their racism: this was a manifestation of the 'African's inability to keep their urges in check'. They falsely believed that the culture of polygamy and widespread promiscuity were baked into local African values and this was the inevitable consequence. This epidemic was ugly, they reasoned, but we simply had to accept it.

These attitudes, to varying degrees, rubbed off on us medical students. Some of us found inspiration in the ethical resistance and fiery opposition that we witnessed. Others found solace in the ugly cynicism, and with it, an excuse to maintain a cool distance between the sterility of the theory and the messiness of the practice of medicine. Some simply remained apolitical, reasoning that this wasn't their fight and they could only do their best with the tools they were given.

It was a turbulent and confusing time for everyone. The stigma was very real and privacy so hard to come by in the packed wards that we didn't even refer to HIV by its name. Instead, ward rounds were filled with euphemisms such as 'retroviral disease', 'RVD', or 'High Five'. When clerking a new patient, we would take a full history and then glance furtively around before dropping our voices and asking, 'By the way ... do you know your HIV status?'

Fear bled into everything. Even minor procedures like drawing blood became fraught with worry about the possibility of a needle-stick injury and possible disease transmission. Urban legends of friends of colleagues who had become HIV-positive in the line of duty sprouted like weeds through concrete. While the wards still had all the usual pathology of adulthood (heart disease, strokes, cancer), these felt completely sidelined by the pandemic-whose-name-we-could-not-publicly-mention. It was made even worse when we had to tell patients they had tested positive. No matter how we dressed it up, no matter how we tried to stay optimistic, the air was heavy with the knowledge that we had just pronounced a death sentence, and a painful one at that.

I watched a young man not much older than me slowly dying – his body covered in the dark splotches of Kaposi's sarcoma, his throat ravaged by yeast, his lungs full of tuberculosis – and wondering what I could do to help him. I could see he was in serious pain so I offered to get the doctor in charge to turn up his morphine infusion. When he saw me stand up and move to leave the room, he gripped my arm and asked me not to leave. 'But I need to get the doctor for the morphine,' I replied.

'You being here is better than morphine,' he whispered.

No lecture had prepared me for this. No one had counselled me on how to comfort someone who was dying. Or what to say to someone who was in such pain and distress. I had studied the pharmacological approach to pain management, but not how to deal with loneliness, fear and sadness. Nor how to manage my own feelings around a patient who was slipping away.

I didn't know what to do or say. In the face of death, words felt impotent and inadequate. What could possibly make sense of it all? But what I did know was that when I had felt spiritually alone the previous year, the presence of another human being was far more comforting than the numbing sensation of drugs. So I stayed.

The man's breathing changed and when he held out his hand, I took it.

I don't know how long I held onto it, but at some point his grip loosened and it turned cold. His eyes developed a faraway look and his breathing became shallower. When I looked up, he was still.

I wished I had done more. I wished I had known what to say or do to comfort him in his final moments. I wished I had been better and that he could have died a more dignified death. He didn't die alone. But he deserved better.

The outrage and grief came to a head when a huge protest march through the streets of Cape Town was organised by the Treatment Action Campaign (TAC) to demand access to antiretroviral treatments. The march included clergy, members of the public, healthcare professionals and some opportunistic politicians. Around 20 000 people took part in the march, demanding that the government stop dragging its heels and honour the order handed down by the court to provide therapy. The march itself was peaceful, but there was a sense of purpose and unity that I found inspiring, even if it was clear that when it came to protests, middle-class white people in South Africa were not exactly versed in the language of defiance. Chants of 'Ho-ho, hey-hey, treatment today!' were effective enough, but attempts by some long-haired, hippie-looking dudes at 'Kumbaya' were more embarrassing than impactful.

The protest, while not massive, garnered international attention. Images of members of the clergy and doctors and civil leaders all united in furious condemnation of government inaction was broadcast on every major news network around the world. Of all the things the ANC government hated, being embarrassed on the world stage was near the top of its list. It sulked for a little while, pretended the march never happened and then grudgingly acknowledged that the roll-out had been 'suboptimal', but that it was still committed to it. The tide shifted subtly but perceptibly against Mbeki, who stopped his public pronouncements and went into a protracted sulk. The TAC and other civic organisations continued their tireless work, and a few years later the ANC began to roll out what has since become the world's largest and most successful antiretroviral programme.

We'll never know how much or how little an impact our march had on the roll-out, but just once it felt good to be roaring our disapproval instead of cynically complaining behind tea-room walls.

The first time I entered a paediatric ward, nothing special happened. Nor was I expecting it to. I had no intention of becoming a paediatrician. Adult general medicine, with its complexities, academia and nerdy pontificating about the causes of electrolyte abnormalities, was where my heart lay. Children were confusing, unpredictable and impenetrable. Unless they were older, they were hopeless at communicating. At best, they belatedly tolerated the presence of healthcare workers. At worst, they screamed bloody murder when you even approached them, regardless of the benevolence of your intentions. Examining them required a patience and flexibility I simply did not possess at the time. They could never be trusted to stay still, let alone inhale on command, or perform complex instructions properly to assess heart sounds. They breathed too rapidly, their hearts beat too quickly to discern the minutiae of murmurs and clicks and they had no necks to look for jugular waves. Their hands gripped and pulled the stethoscope while I was listening to their chests, which hurt my ears but seemed to bring them great amusement.

They were also a nightmare for procedures. Whereas adults would sit patiently while you stabbed their arm for the third time trying to get blood, children howled and wailed and squirmed and writhed. Whereas drains and lines would stay in adults for days, the drips and tubes we used in children, with their tiny lumens and delicate secures, were often quickly dislodged, either by accident or design, by children who simply had better things to do than tolerate their presence.

And then came Sipho.

Sipho was a severely malnourished child who looked like a wizened old man when he arrived. Except he was only nine months old. The skin sagged off his body tiredly and his lips and tongue were cracked and swollen from iron deficiency. Sores and ulcers covered most of his arms and legs. What little moisture he had in his body seemed to be expelled by the constant tears that spilled out of his eyes.

His mother was unemployed and had been abandoned by her partner. Due to losing her ID card, she was unable to access the government's child-support grant. She had TB and was skin and bones herself. Her tired, chronically ill body was unable to produce the milk needed to breastfeed Sipho. She and her three other children lived with her mother in a shack in Khayelitsha, and survived on her pension, which was just over R300 a month at the time.

In desperation to feed Sipho, she had started making mealie meal and siphoning off the water at the top to use as a milk substitute.

She had also tried giving him pap as a solid food, but this wasn't enough. Sipho was wasting away, and this seemed to have the same effect on her, as if her failure to feed her son was her fault, and enduring starvation was her penance. She was too ashamed to seek help and wouldn't have known where to go even if she wanted it.

Eventually, one night, Sipho started to cry. And he would not stop. Neither water, nor food, nor gentle rocking would comfort him. One of the neighbours, who got tired of the howls, offered to give Sipho's mother taxi money to get to the hospital. Sipho screamed the entire journey.

He cried when we took bloods and put up an IV line to rehydrate him. He cried when we put a tube into his stomach to help feed him. He cried when we tried to comfort him and he cried when we left him alone. His enormous brown eyes, which felt like they were sizing up your very soul, contained a never-ending well of tears. He even cried in his sleep, with tears squeezing from his eyes when he eventually nodded off.

Sipho never stopped crying, but he did start gaining weight. The creams we rubbed onto his dry skin started to ease the weeping sores, the vitamins and iron we gave him helped his cracked lips to heal and gave him more energy. Which he used to cry even louder. In fact, only one thing stopped Sipho from crying.

Me.

I'm still not sure why. I didn't do anything discernibly different from any of my colleagues. If anything, I was more awkward around him than they were, feeling that I lacked the intrinsic understanding some seemed to possess around children. I remember feeling jealous at how smoothly some of my colleagues handled kids, scooping them up, swaddling them, nursing them with practised ease. Whereas my movements felt awkward and robotic, like I was handling a ticking bomb. But when Sipho sat in my lap, for a few brief, blissful minutes there was (golden) silence in the ward. Maybe it was my thick curly hair that he enjoyed tugging. Maybe it was my big nose, whose nostrils he enjoyed excavating with his finger. Maybe it was that he appeared to be a big fan of hard rock. Once, while soothing him, I started playing 'Monkey Wrench' by the Foo Fighters on my Discman, and when the first crunching riff started, he paused, looked at me confusedly and then promptly fell asleep. He only woke up and resumed crying when the music stopped, but nodded off again when 'Everlong' got to the loud part.

Maybe it was the head scratches. His brittle, patchy hair had fallen out in clumps, but he was particularly amenable to having the remaining areas gently scratched.

Maybe it was the philosophical conversations I had with him about life, love and the universe. He scrunched his forehead up as I regaled him with stories about the current political landscape or the latest celebrity scandal. He would raise a quizzical brow when I complained about work that my sponsor was making me complete, or how trite I occasionally found the slogans at AA meetings.

I don't think that Sipho loved me. He hardly smiled, nor was he ever very affectionate. But in a world of malnourishment and pain, he tolerated me, which was a step up from almost everyone else. His mother, too, was growing more robust once her TB medication started kicking in. She had gained some weight and the hollowness of her cheeks began filling out. She, too, seemed not to mind my presence and affectionately called me the 'stylish doctor' one day after seeing me wearing a pink shirt. This comment was hilarious to everyone in the ward because never before, or since, have I been accused of being 'stylish'.

I remember saying goodbye to Sipho when my block ended. He looked me over, appeared to understand, and for the first time in the few weeks I had cradled him, he cried.

About a month later, while doing some administrative work, I found myself back in the paediatric hospital. I decided to pay Sipho a visit.

Sitting in his bed was a different child. I panicked. It was far too soon for Sipho to have been discharged. If someone else was in his bed this could only mean he had been moved elsewhere because of a deterioration or – God forbid – that he had died.

I looked a little closer. This young boy was healthy, with a clear layer of fat under his skin and a sheen of moisturiser over his body. He was engrossed with a toy, which he was alternately putting in his mouth and then waving chaotically in front of his face. It was only when he looked at me that I recognised the brown eyes. I couldn't believe it. It was Sipho.

'He's better now, eh, Doctor?' I turned towards the voice and almost gasped. Sipho's mother, too, was completely different. Her broken frame seemed, if not completely repaired, at least on the mend. Her voice no longer whispered, but projected calmness and warmth. I found out that once she started to feel better on the medication, she had managed to get a replacement ID from Home Affairs. With this she had been able to access the child-support grant for Sipho. Her appetite had improved and the nourishment we had been giving her boy had fed her soul as well. She was hoping, once he was discharged, to begin looking for a job. Her old employers were even considering rehiring her.

She glanced down. For the first time, her voice cracked. 'You helped fix him.'

'Me? Oh god, no. It was the whole team. The doctors and nurses and social workers. I'm just a student trying to learn.'

'Yes. I am grateful to all of them. But he chose you. You were the one who made him feel better; feel safe. He even liked your loud, ugly music. I don't know why. Everyone else in the ward hated it. But it calmed him.'

I didn't really know what to say. I mumbled something and then Sipho pointed at me and did something I had never seen him do before. He smiled.

In between classes and the hospital, I was also working hard to maintain my sobriety. This meant attending at least three AA or NA meetings every week. I had taken my sponsor's advice to get involved in service and volunteered to be the treasurer at my home group. Usually, you had to be at least a year clean and sober to be considered for the role, but my predecessor had relapsed and taken all the group's funds with him, and there were no other volunteers, so beggars couldn't be choosers. It was strange hopping from a busy day at the hospital, where I was tending to the sick and needy, to meetings where I was simply another recovering addict or alcoholic. In one environment, I was the (trainee) healer: the smart medical student who needed to project calmness, intelligence and control. In another I was the chaotic (recovering) addict: hanging out with other chaotic (recovering) addicts and using that chaos as a blueprint towards finding ongoing peace and sobriety. In neither environment was I allowed to refer to the other. Colleagues and clinicians at work couldn't know anything about my 'issue' because it would show that I was defective, weak and not resilient enough for this job. Mental illness – and addiction in particular – were not spoken about publicly in the medical field. Any hint of an impediment could go on your record and follow you for the rest of your days, limiting career prospects and even registration with licensing bodies. Best to keep your problems to yourself. Got personal issues gnawing at you? Walk them off, put a smile on that face and get back to your patients. Doctors were supposed to have it together. We were supposed to be confident and in control. After all, when you're at your lowest ebb, having the worst day of your life, you want calm assurance from your carer, not messy and human frailty. Exhibiting weakness would damage both our colleagues' and patients' trust in our judgement. My past potentially dented and scratched the shiny, bulletproof façade that patients relied upon in their time of need. When I was asked what I had been doing the past year, I tried my best to walk the line between lying (which I wanted to avoid) and total and honest disclosure. I'd usually mumble something about 'personal issues' and rapidly change the subject.

This need to conceal a part of myself occurred in my recovery, too. Twelve-step programmes pride themselves on anonymity. At meetings, none of us are defined by our jobs or status. Like everyone else in the room, I was just another addict seeking recovery. Declaring myself to be a medical student would have been regarded as boastful and disrespectful. At least that's what I told myself at the time. More likely, I wanted to preserve the fragile identity I had rebuilt for myself, that of the self-assured trainee doctor. Despite doing the hard work, getting my life together, and hitting one entire year sober, I still carried heaps of shame around with me. There was a pervasive fear that a patient, or a patient's family member, might identify me from a meeting, or that I would be 'outed' if I revealed too much of my professional life and struggles to a bunch of strangers. While the programmes discourage gossip about individual people, preferring to focus on 'principles', I knew as well as anyone else that news flies around the recovery circles. As a result, my career was something I kept resolutely to myself. But it meant that when I was asked to share, there was a large chunk of my life I had to try to figure out alone.

One day my sponsor called me on it. 'Why do you never talk about the stuff at hospital, Al? I'm not referring to confidential shit but about how you're feeling and what it's like going back and being around patients again? You must be feeling *all* the fucking emotions right now, except this time you can't drink them away. So why not talk about them?'

'Mate, I can't. I can't tell people I'm a med student. What would they think?' I whined.

He exhaled loudly. 'Jee-zuz. You have some humility to learn, my guy. You think you're the only "important" person at those meetings? What if I told you that within our circle there's one of Cape Town's top commercial lawyers? Guy used to drive a Lamborghini before he wrapped it around a tree one night in a drunken stupor. Know that guy who shared tonight on struggling to find creativity in recovery? That's one of the most eminent architects in the country. You need to get over yourself and share what's really going on.'

'Easy for you to say. You work as a mechanic. No one cares if you go to AA meetings or not.' I was shocked at what I had just said and would have done anything to recover the hurtful words I had so carelessly sprayed in his direction.

'God. I'm so sorry. What an awful thing to say. Please let me make it up to you.'

A flicker of hurt crossed his face before his trademark amusedly philosophical look returned. I had always found it remarkable how he managed to be deeply serious and deviously cheeky at the same time. 'I think I know how.'

'Yeah? How?'

'You're going to be the main sharer at our next meeting. And you're going to talk about what happens at work. You don't have to be specific. You don't even have to mention what kind of work you do. But I want you to talk about how all the stuff you experience makes you feel. And how you stay sober, regardless.'

And so, the following week, for twenty minutes, a group of strangers listened to my story. I tried to keep it as real as possible while emphasising the struggles I still encountered.

I spoke about the loneliness of being the only recovering addict in my class. The sadness at being without my original group of school and university friends who had graduated and either gone to Johannesburg or London to begin their jobs and new lives. The shame and judgement I still felt whenever someone laughed or looked in my direction, convinced I was being gossiped about and mocked. But I also spoke about the joy I had felt reconnecting with patients, and about how my woundedness had seemed to, paradoxically, bring me closer to them. It was as if they could sense, without being told, that I was more like them than some other physicians. That I knew what it was like on the other end of a stethoscope.

When people were sharing back, an old-timer with thirty years of sobriety under his belt leaned forward and said, 'I wish more of my doctors were in recovery! Maybe then they'd actually listen to me!' He chuckled but a wave of appreciative and agreeing nods rippled around the group. It was around that time that I decided that I would be more honest about who I was. People seemed to think it helped them. But really it helped me, too.

'Shit, that's a bad injury.' I was roused from my semi-nap by the voice of the surgical registrar. It was 3am and we were at the admissions desk. I was three weeks into my surgical rotation and, by now, had lost all semblance of a normal sleeping routine. Days bled into each other and I couldn't remember the last time I had felt fully refreshed.

The emergency department had called. A young man in his early twenties had come off his motorcycle an hour before. He had multiple injuries, but, crucially, his head was unharmed ('Thank fuck for helmets,' I remember hearing someone mutter). The biggest problem was his arm. In landing on it at such high speed, he had nearly ripped it clean off from the shoulder joint. There was extensive damage, but the real concern was the blood supply. The major vessels nourishing his arm had been badly damaged and the tissue was dying. He needed emergency surgery. Tonight.

The registrar didn't even need to see the patient to know that he was out of his depth, and this meant having to call the consultant in to assist. He gulped and picked up the phone. Ten minutes later, Dr Ashwari arrived.

His reputation, like a hot breeze, seemed to pre-empt his arrival. He was all compact energy and intense focus. An excellent surgeon, he didn't suffer fools. He was also a gross misogynist. More than once he had stated outright that female medical students would do better in their oral exams if they arrived in short skirts. He also insinuated, in many ways, that surgery was no place for women. Once on a ward round, when told that a female registrar was on maternity leave, he had sighed theatrically and said he wished the women would be more considerate and 'plan' their pregnancies so as not to disrupt patient care. In a journal club earlier in the week (where some hapless registrar had to analyse a study and then have that analysis scrutinised by the entire staff), an intern had suggested using a different type of suturing material to the type commonly used to close an internal wound.

'And what may I ask is the evidence for this claim?' Dr Ashwari had asked, his voice flying like a dart from the back of the room.

'Well, uh, I read about it in this article ...'

'So is your claim based on a well-conducted randomised control trial published in a reputable journal?'

'Well ... no ... but ...'

'So, what's it based on?' The silence that followed swallowed the room.

'I ... uh ... read about it in a magazine ...'

'A *magazine*?! Boy, I didn't know *People* had become an authority on surgical techniques! Look here, young man. In this department we go by evidence. And I mean *good* evidence. Level-1 stuff. Not pie-in-the-sky opinions from people you wouldn't want operating on your grandmother. Is that understood?' He settled back in his chair. No further suggestions were made during that journal club.

The patient was prepped and rushed to theatre. Dr Ashwari, myself and the registrar all scrubbed in. Dr Ashwari and the registrar would be operating, while I observed. The hierarchy in surgery was among the strictest I had ever observed. I recalled that on our first day of the surgery rotation one of the senior consultants had stood in front of us and said, 'Okay, young gentlemen and ladies. Surgery is tough. If you're too busy worrying about make-up, or having babies, then this probably isn't the rotation for you. I know this generation of med students likes to complain a lot, but truth be told I don't want to hear it. It's a privilege to be here and you should all be grateful for the opportunity. You'll see more surgery in the next few weeks than international trainees see in their entirety of med school. If you have any questions, please ask your intern. If the intern doesn't know, they'll ask the medical officer. If the medical officer doesn't know, they'll ask the registrar. If the registrar doesn't know, they'll ask the consultant. If the *consultant* doesn't know, they'll ask God.' Here he paused. 'And if *God* doesn't know ... well ... he'll ask me.' The glint in his eye and the tiny smirk had let us all know that he was joking ... but only a little. The point remained that, in surgery, the pecking order is rigid; there is no room for doubt or insecurity. If you can't handle it, step aside for someone else who can.

The hiss of the ventilator brought me back to the moment. The anaesthetist had swiftly and delicately put the patient under, intubated him and attached him to the ventilator. When we finally undressed the bandage over his shoulder, we realised the Herculean task that lay ahead. The joint was a mangled mess and I wasn't sure how *anyone* could even begin to fix it. Dr Ashwari, undaunted, started meticulously correcting the damage. Blood vessels I didn't even know existed were lovingly identified and sewn back together with the deftest of touches. It was slow going but it was incredible to behold. I felt like I was in the presence of a maestro. Practised hands dissected and isolated and repaired. Five hours went by, and it was clear that we still had a long way to go. The hot lights had started to take their toll, however, and both Dr Ashwari and the registrar were drenched in sweat. The patient was stable so a time-out was called.

The registrar leaned over to me and said that he could feel his blood sugar levels were low. Would I mind grabbing something for him from the vending machine? I de-gowned and scuttled out, but the only item left in the dejected-looking machine was an ancient packet of jelly babies. It accepted my money and I returned to the theatre door where the registrar had poked his head out. He was still sterile and looking a bit faint, so I found a way of inserting the jelly babies into his mouth through the side of his mask. He gobbled them gratefully and I could see the colour return to his cheeks as his blood sugar rose. He perked up instantly, and by the time I had re-scrubbed and joined him at the table, he was visibly more animated.

We were alone with the patient. Dr Ashwari was in the corner of the theatre, conversing with the anaesthetist about how best to maintain the patient's blood pressure for the rest of the operation, and the scrub nurse was a few metres away checking the gauze bandages. The registrar was leaning over the exposed shoulder inspecting Dr Ashwari's handiwork when the unthinkable happened.

It's a cliché in the movies that disasters occur in slow motion, but that's exactly what happened. As he tilted his mask over the surgical site, a single, renegade jelly baby, nestled somewhere undetected in his mask, rolled towards the end of the material above his nose, teetered precipitously and then slipped out.

The registrar later told me that in the period it took for the jelly baby to fall from his mask directly into the patient's shoulder cavity, his entire medical career flashed before his eyes. This case was Dr Ashwari's masterpiece, destroyed in a second by a ruinous jelly baby disrupting the sterile field. There would be shouting, there would be gesticulating. There would be admonishments and threats, but there would be no forgiveness. Surgeons have long memories and cruel WhatsApp groups. Mistakes and bad outcomes were mercilessly dissected and analysed. A few years earlier a surgeon had accidentally sewn a medical student's gown to a patient while closing. Another had set a patient on fire when they used the electrical scalpel (diathermy) on a patient's skin before the alcohol cleaning agent had fully evaporated. I don't think either of them ever lived those down.

This mistake was potentially career-ending and we both knew it. The registrar's eyes met mine and all I could see was unbridled panic. But there was something else, too. A silent plea, to help a colleague. In this situation, I suddenly had the power. I could alert Dr Ashwari; I could do nothing; or I could help. I looked back and nodded imperceptibly. We only had a few seconds at most before either Dr Ashwari or the scrub nurse returned. We both started rummaging through the wound desperately trying to find the jelly baby while trying to avoid the delicate surgical work. Every time we spotted it, it slipped through our fingers and fell deeper into the cavernous wound. Navigating the nerves and arteries made me grateful, perhaps for the first time, that I had paid attention in anatomy class. After a few seconds, we heard Dr Ashwari returning to the table. I knew what I needed to do: run interference.

I stepped back. 'Soooooooo! Dr Ashwari! What an absolutely *fascinating* case this is, but I'm really struggling with my brachial

PART 2: THE HISTORY

plexus anatomy. I know it's early but could you just go through it again with me?'

Dr Ashwari eyed me suspiciously. 'Did you not pay attention during your anatomy lectures? I don't think we have time for this.' He began shuffling past me. I decided it was time to bring out the big guns: flattery and competition.

'Oh, absolutely! It's just ... I was in theatre with Dr Boyer the other day and he said the right inferior thyroid vein joins the right innominate vein. But I could have sworn you told us it joins the left innominate vein. He seemed pretty adamant ...'

Dr Ashwari stopped. 'Oh for goodness' sake. Medicine is going to the dogs.' And he proceeded to verbally map out the vascular anatomy of the shoulder and chest in excruciating detail.

All the while, I was keeping an eye on the registrar. After about forty-five seconds, he let out a grunt and I saw him holding the bloodied jelly baby in his fingers. When Dr Ashwari finished discussing anatomy with me and returned to the wound, the registrar casually remarked, 'Gosh, it's quite a dirty wound isn't it? We really should irrigate it thoroughly and start some broad-spectrum antibiotics ...'

Three hours later we emerged. The remainder of the surgery had gone well. We had saved the blood supply to the arm and the neurosurgeons were fixing his nerves. When we got out of theatre, the registrar beckoned me over.

'Thanks, Alastair. You saved me twice in there. I get very low blood sugar sometimes but I don't tell anyone because they would think I was needlessly complaining. I would appreciate it if you kept this, ah, "episode" to yourself?' I nodded.

'Now ... what are we going to do about this?' He had put the bloodied jelly baby in a specimen jar and was holding it up.

'Throw it away?' I offered.

'Nah. If he gets an infection we need to know how best to treat him.'

'Should we send it to the lab?' I said.

'I don't know! Do labs do tests on jelly babies? How would we explain it?'

'Just send it anyway and see what comes back.'

I scribbled some notes on a requisition chart, he signed it, and the jelly baby disappeared into the bowels of the hospital.

A few days later, the report was ready. The microbiologist personally called me. 'Why is this jelly baby covered in blood?'

'Do you really want to know?'

'You know what? On second thought, I don't. There's no way there's an answer to that that will improve my day. Life's too short.' The report showed, unsurprisingly, 'multiple organisms'. These included a streptococcus notorious for being 'flesh-eating'. Dr Ashwari barely raised an eyelid when we recommended broadening the patient's antibiotics further on the next ward round.

By the end of fourth year, I had definitively decided that I wanted to pursue a career in adult internal medicine. While I had enjoyed my time in the other specialties, internal medicine seemed the most cerebral and therefore the best fit for me. Obstetrics and gynaecology involved too much blood and amniotic fluid. The episode with Dr Ashwari and the jelly baby had shown me how competitive, yet fragile, the surgical path could be, and how easily everything could come undone in a few chaotic seconds. When I hadn't been rummaging for errant jelly babies, surgery had involved a lot of standing under hot lights, rigorously retracting organs and watching the surgeon spend ninety per cent of their time doing their best to avoid hitting important blood vessels. If your concentration slipped for even one moment and you relaxed your

PART 2: THE HISTORY

grip, compromising the surgeon's field of vision, they would let you know *all* about it. More than one student found the bright lights, heat and heavy surgical gowns so overwhelming that they clean fainted. As long as you didn't contaminate the sterile surgical field while crashing down, the surgeons usually didn't take any notice and simply carried on without you.

There were students in the class who seemed designed for surgery, however. They delighted in the aura that surgeons have around them; a sense that having dissected living humans to their very essence, they had seen something the rest of us hadn't. Surgery was *important*. Surgeons on a ward round were *important*. Time *was* of the essence. Extensive and unnecessary notes wasted time and therefore endangered patients. Even in their clipped state, notes seemed *important*:

58y.o. ♂, D4 post ø,
Lap app ruptured App
S: Feeling better O: No concerns
Normal labs, apyrexial, pt. PU√, PSx, TF PO
P: Cont. Mx, Stop abx, mobilize

The simple fact was that surgery was where the cool kids went. And I have never been cool in my life.

Internal medicine, on the other hand, felt a lot nerdier, which suited me fine. Unkempt physicians whose hair hadn't seen a hairbrush in weeks shuffled around, and we spent hours discussing the minutiae of every case. We detoured through the peaks and valleys of electrolyte abnormalities, fluid balance and pathophysiology. We hacked our way through the forests of autoimmune disease and sepsis management. A good differential diagnosis list meant the difference between effulgent praise and a stern silence. In short, it felt like home. Or, at least, home for my brain. The patients themselves, while never treated unkindly, were often excluded from the complex conversations that took place around them. Rarely did we ask how it felt to have fifteen sets of strange eyes scanning their bodies. Or whether there was something dehumanising about having their most personal details shared so widely among a large group. In a country where black bodies had traditionally been exploited and disregarded, especially by white people, this felt even more uncomfortable.

This was also where a racial tension among the trainees began to take root. During one round, a cardiology professor asked a black student to listen to the heart and tell him what she heard. After doing a thorough cardiac exam and listening intently, she informed him that she heard a systolic murmur caused by turbulence in the heart from a regurgitant valve. The professor asked her to time it and after listening for a few more seconds, she proudly said, 'Two seconds.'

There was a tittering in the group and an exchange of slightly exasperated smiles. A subtle but visible rolling of the eyes. She had misunderstood the question. The professor had not meant for her to time the heart rate, but to time where in the cardiac cycle the murmur was occurring; he wanted her to tell him if it was a pansystolic or ejection systolic murmur.

'It's okay, young lady,' the professor murmured. 'Some of us take longer to hear these things than others.'

Within the group, I heard a whisper, 'This is what happens when you let all these affirmatives in,' referring to the university's policy of affirmative action.

I have no idea if she heard that remark, but even from a few feet away, I could feel the redness climbing up her cheeks. She managed, through some superhuman effort, not to cry, but I could feel that she was close. The thing was, she knew exactly how to time a murmur. I had seen her do it many times. But English was her third language, and she had, in the stress of the moment, misunderstood the subtleties of what was being asked of her. It was unfair for people to giggle, especially when similar mistakes made by white students never received the same level of scrutiny. During the same round, under stress, a white student had percussed for the spleen on the wrong side of the body. The round stayed quiet. Mean remarks about the suitability of the student's place in the class were barely raised for white students.

None of this was overt and if an accusation of racism had been made against anyone on that round, there would have been fulsome and angry denials. But Groote Schuur Hospital had a wretched history of racism. During apartheid, patients were separated into different wards based on their skin colour. Some doctors refused to see black patients and the care those patients had received was markedly inferior to their white counterparts. In those days, black doctors and medical students were very rare. It was impossible to shake the notion that despite the excitement of the 'Rainbow Nation' and the fuzzy feeling Nelson Mandela had recently imparted, racism was baked into the foundation of the hospital, into the foundation of our class, and that everyone was simply too polite to say anything.

Eventually, it all boiled over. A group of students claimed that one of the departments was discriminating against them because of their race. They alleged that tests written by white students were being graded less harshly than those written by black students. This was a very difficult allegation to prove, because, in theory, tests were anonymous. In reality, the groups were small, and due to the number of assignments we submitted, examiners became very familiar with everyone's handwriting and knew exactly who they were grading.

The department angrily denied the allegations but they became hard to ignore because they were coming from some very bright students who were passing comfortably and had little reason to lie. Many of the white students were bemused. We had no inkling that there was this much anger. Our experiences had largely been positive so it took us by surprise that the lens through which we viewed medical school was not a universal one.

The truth was that our skin colour *had* played a huge role in how we experienced medical school in South Africa. While there will always be differences in any large group of new students anywhere, with some benefiting from wealth and privilege and others struggling against hardship and adversity, in our class this disparity was both magnified and predictable. If you were white, the system had generally tilted in your favour. If you were not, you usually had a host of obstacles to overcome.

As a young white man, I had been exceedingly well prepared for university by the private school I attended. The classes were all in my first language, English. I could afford to buy all the necessary textbooks and additional ones too. I had a car, which meant I could get around easily, and I did not need to work to support myself through medical school. When I was crippled by addiction, I had the funds and the support networks to help me get sober. In contrast, thanks to apartheid, most of my black counterparts had gone to poorly funded, often rural public schools, lacking in many basic amenities. English was often their third, or even fourth language, and while they spoke it beautifully, they sometimes lacked the ability to parse the nuances and subtleties that come from conversing in your mother tongue. The textbooks were often too expensive to afford, which meant they had to use the copies in the library, which didn't have enough supply to meet the demand. Many did not have cars so they had to get up earlier to catch the university shuttles. To afford their fees, most worked additional jobs, which ate into their study time. On top of this, they found themselves occupying a space which, until recently, they had been cruelly excluded from. I can only imagine what it must have felt like to wander past the photos of the previous deans of the university in the library and not see a single face of colour. Or to peruse the pictures of previous classes, which were more than ninety-five per cent white, in a country that was overwhelmingly black. Or to gaze upon the statue of someone who had viciously oppressed their ancestors, occupying pride of place in the centre of the campus. When I first walked into medical school, I felt like I belonged; when many black students did, they felt that they were unwelcome visitors in a hostile land.

The allegations of racism were never fully resolved, but the university endeavoured to be more transparent in how it marked papers. But the situation highlighted one key point: the wounds of the past still lingered. While they may have been unnoticeable to some of us, there were others who keenly felt the raw pain and anguish.

In our final year we had to decide where we wanted to do the mandatory two-year internship after we (hopefully) graduated. Those final months of medical school were when the excitement really began to ramp up. After six years of study (in my case, seven), we were ready to embrace a new challenge. We were tired of endless tests and exams and oral quizzes and being at the bottom of the medical hierarchy. We were ready for the next step and, finally, a salary.

The mechanics of getting an internship spot at a desired hospital were complex in conception and labyrinthine in execution. Students listed five possible hospitals they were prepared to work at, with emphasis on the all-important 'first choice'. If your medical school was assigned, say, five posts at a particular hospital and ten people put that as their first choice, all the names would go into a hat and the first five drawn would be considered successful. If you didn't get your first choice, you had to wait until all the first-choicers had been placed before settling for the dregs of the remaining hospitals. If you were unsuccessful with all your choices, you were placed somewhere randomly (usually very rural).

Unsurprisingly, hospitals in Cape Town were at a premium because most of the class was either from Cape Town or had settled there and didn't feel like relocating their whole lives again. Many had partners or spouses or sick family members who they did not want to move away from. Many found the process unbearably stressful and destabilising.

I was not one of them.

From early on, I decided to pick Chris Hani Baragwanath. Given its sheer size, it was allocated twelve spots at our medical school. Because of its fearsome reputation, in any given year, it never came close to filling all of them. As a result, I knew that if I put it as my first choice, I would get it. All my fellow students knew this, too, and Bara was so desperate to get its interns that people were told definitively *not* to write it as one of their five choices if they didn't want to go there.

'You put Bara *anywhere* on your list, you get Bara. Simple as that,' was a common refrain, meant mostly as a warning for the unwary or those foolish enough to include it as a 'back-up' to fill the slots on their application.

The reason I chose Bara was precisely the reason so many avoided it: I wanted to experience the harshest test internship could throw my way. Baragwanath was regarded as the 'Navy SEALs' of internship; a stern challenge that, like a forge, would either shape you into a sturdier version of yourself or break you in the process.

PART 2: THE HISTORY

I wanted to be the best, most competent physician I could, which meant I had to be able to withstand the worst of what public South African hospitals could throw my way. I needed to know, in my heart, that I had it in me. I also wanted to make a difference.

There was a joke that those who stayed at Groote Schuur did so little of consequence and were given such limited responsibility that they were simply glorified porters; that the title of our degree (MBChB) instead of meaning 'Bachelor of Medicine and Surgery', instead stood for 'Messenger Boy, Carrier of Human Blood'. While this was harsh, and often untrue (interns at Groote Schuur work very hard), I wanted to work somewhere where I was making a difference to people's lives, even as an intern.

There was another reason I chose Baragwanath. I was ready for a change. Cape Town can sometimes feel small and I was feeling stagnant. The same faces in the AA meetings, the same clinicians in the hospitals. I was ready for Big Bad Johannesburg.

And so it came time for graduation and the fulfilment of many years of hard work. Graduation took place in the former 'Great Hall' of UCT (now the Sarah Baartman Hall). Everyone who went up on that stage had sweated blood and tears to earn the degree and thoroughly earned the riotous applause and ululations that greeted them. We had all laboured over our textbooks long into the night. We had missed parties, birthdays and anniversaries because of our academic responsibilities. We had watched our friends start their jobs and careers while we remained penniless students. As I took the steps onto the stage, I remembered how just a few years before, I had been told I was no longer welcome on campus because of my drinking. Now, I was over three years sober and graduating with distinction. It was a private satisfaction, but I knew that I was only there because of the countless hands that had lifted me up:

my counsellors, my sponsor and the thousands of people who had humbled themselves and sat in AA meetings so that I could join them. But I had also put in the work. A thousand times I had ordered a Coke when I could have ordered a beer. A thousand times I had taken myself to a meeting when I could have stayed at home. A thousand times I opted to share my shit and put myself in a position of vulnerability rather than stay quiet. I was walking onto that stage because, for over a thousand days, through some alchemic miracle, I had not taken any alcohol into my body despite drinking being my default state.

I had earned this moment of satisfaction. One momentous journey was ending. I thought I knew where the next one was heading. I couldn't have been more wrong.

PART 3
The Prescription

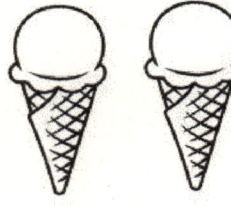

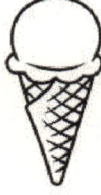

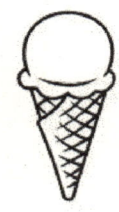

PART 3

The Prescription

Chapter 12
WITNESSING JASON'S JOURNEY

'He's not going to make it. Call palliative care.' The instruction was given in a neutral tone, as if asking us to book a chest X-ray or get a dietetics opinion. The intern, new to the ward and unfamiliar with the patient, diligently recorded the consultant's instruction on the patient list and eagerly looked up, awaiting the next one. I exhaled sharply with relief. I had been the registrar looking after the boy in the bed in front of us for over four weeks, and I was at my wits' end.

Jason was a seven-year-old boy who had a metabolic condition that caused a slow degeneration of his brain and central nervous system. There are different variations of this disease, some more treatable than others. While we were figuring out which type he had, Jason had been transferred to the paediatric ICU at the hospital where I was doing my paediatric registrar time. It was here that I first encountered him.

From the beginning, managing Jason was a challenge. To attempt to properly diagnose him, Jason had undergone numerous and painful tests. His bed was surrounded by concerned-looking neurologists, perplexed metabolic experts and increasingly exasperated pain management teams. Distressingly, whatever the condition was, it was hurting him. His nerves were degenerating and misfiring slowly, which left him in constant pain that was becoming harder and harder to manage. His mother sat diligently and quietly by Jason's bedside, giving the teams of doctors and healthcare workers their space, occasionally placing her hand tenderly on her son's forehead when she had a few precious moments alone with him.

Because no one knew Jason's underlying issue, or what condition he had, he was kept on 'full intervention' while we worked to properly diagnose him. This meant that everything that was needed to keep him alive, no matter how invasive or painful, was on the table. If he arrested, for whatever reason, he would be fully resuscitated, with no effort spared in the attempt to save him.

The hope was that we would discover that he had something that was reversible. But as time went on, those of us who were caring for him every day realised that this was very unlikely. The tests may have been equivocal, but messages from Jason's own body couldn't have been any clearer: it was shutting down. Trying to prevent this while awaiting the results from even more investigations for rarer and more complicated conditions was becoming harder and harder. He needed multiple IV lines for the fluids to keep him hydrated, administer the medications to manage his pain and provide the constant infusions of anticonvulsants to control the seizures that had recently started and were getting longer and more severe. This told us that the neurones in his brain were now being affected. Meanwhile, his frayed peripheral nerves shot disjointed and painful signals to his spinal cord and brain every time we touched him. The IV lines themselves were deeply uncomfortable, causing him to constantly try to pull them out.

Eventually, when all our investigations came back as negative, Jason was sent down to the general paediatric ward because his prognosis was 'guarded' and PICU needed the bed for a patient whose condition *could* be reversed.

'He clearly has a neurodegenerative condition,' the neurologist sighed. 'It's almost certainly fatal and I'm not sure anything can be done to reverse it. Other than controlling the seizures, there's nothing else we can offer. So we're signing off. We won't be back to see him unless you have any specific questions for us.'

As the days went by, and it became apparent that no satisfactory diagnosis could be found, the specialist teams followed neurology's lead and gradually drifted away. They were polite and helpful, but with nothing to hang their collective hats on, there was little that they felt they could offer.

Jason, meanwhile, continued to deteriorate in the ward and managing him became more and more challenging. One night I was called to reinsert a catheter that had come out. Jason was waiting in the procedure room and the equipment was set up and ready for me. He knew what was coming, but instead of the usual crying and objections, this time he was resigned. Two tear tracks were drying down each of his cheeks and he was doing his best to stifle his sobs. His mother was holding his hand and singing a soothing lullaby into his ear.

At that moment, I knew there had to be a better way.

Jason was surrounded by hard-working, kind and diligent people who all wanted what was best for him, but it wasn't working. We were making him miserable. So when the consultant suggested we contact the palliative care team, I was both relieved and confused.

'I didn't know the hospital had a palliative care team,' I said after the suggestion was made.

'It's new,' the consultant replied. 'They've managed to find some

PART 3: THE PRESCRIPTION

funding or something. I don't usually like giving up on patients, but have you got any better ideas?'

I confessed that I didn't and we moved on. When the round was done, the intern made the call.

I was organising the transfer of a patient to the PICU a few hours later when I heard a soft knock on the door. I turned around and saw two women I did not recognise standing in the doorway and smiling. It had not been a 'smiling' type of day, with everyone running around frantically clearing space for the new patients we were expecting, so that immediately piqued my interest and made me take note.

'Hi! Can I help you?' I tried to convey politeness, but also that I was busy and they needed to get on with whatever they had to say.

'We're from PaedsPal,' the slightly older woman said brightly. 'You asked us to come and assess Jason? Well, we have and we're ready to provide some feedback and recommendations.'

'Oh. Great! Thanks. Please come and sit.' I tried to make some room in the cluttered office that was full of outdated treatment algorithms, coffee cups, doughnut boxes and patient notes. The women settled on some chairs and immediately introduced themselves by their first names. The younger one with blonde hair, Lisa, I vaguely recognised from registrar teaching days. She had been completing her time just as I was beginning mine. She was known for her quirky sense of humour and fondness for quoting from the movie *Anchorman*. The slightly older woman, Mary, radiated peace and authority, which is what trainees want from referral services. Lisa began, 'So, Jason. God, what a challenging case. Firstly, Agnes thinks you're amazing and thanks you for being so gentle with her son.'

I blinked. Agnes was Jason's mother. I had tried to comfort her as best I could during the ordeal, but always felt I had failed miserably.

Hearing that she was grateful threw me off a bit. I also wasn't sure what this had to do with Jason's palliative management. 'Uh ... thanks. I'm so sorry she has to go through all of this.'

'Since we're talking about Agnes,' Lisa continued, 'we really need to get her additional support. She was fired from her job as a cleaner because she spends so much time here at the hospital with Jason.'

I was ashamed to admit that I didn't know this.

'Her employer isn't aware of the full story, so we're going to get in contact with him to explain what's going on and ask him to reconsider. Aggie' – I hadn't heard anyone call her that, but it sounded so natural when Lisa said it – 'has been a diligent worker for over twelve years with no disciplinary issues. If her employer won't reconsider, we'll get the social worker to contact the CCMA and see if there's legal recourse.'

I started writing all her comments down, but Mary gently touched me on my arm. 'No need to scribble. We've written it all in our notes with a copy in the file.'

Lisa continued, 'We're also worried about the home situation.'

'Yeah,' I interjected, eager to show that I hadn't ignored Jason's living circumstances entirely. 'There are two other children at home who are being looked after by the neighbours.'

'Right,' said Lisa. 'But this isn't manageable long term. Aggie needs to go home, but she doesn't have the money to constantly be taking taxis back and forth. The taxis have raised their prices what with petrol doing its thing, and she's struggling without a pay cheque.'

I nodded and sighed. These problems seemed insurmountable and I had twenty other kids in my ward who also needed my help. I think Mary could sense my growing despair and jumped in. 'Don't panic. We have connections with the hospital social services who have access to transport funds. If that fails, we also have a small

PART 3: THE PRESCRIPTION

kitty of cash we keep for such emergencies. We'll sort it out.'

I exhaled in relief. After a few more minutes thrashing out solutions for Jason's home situation, we got to Jason himself.

'Jason and his mother both know he's dying and they were wondering when he could go home? He's tired of the drips and the catheters and the tests. He misses his dog.'

I was taken aback. No one I knew had initiated any of these conversations with Jason or Agnes. For a brief moment, I felt angry that these discussions had been conducted without me. 'How do you know?'

'He and Aggie told us. It was one of the first things they said.' Lisa acted as if this were no big deal; as if Jason had just told her who his favourite superhero was. 'Don't get me wrong – they're grateful for the effort everyone has put in, and they're happy to continue if you think he can be cured – but in their hearts they feel like he's never going to recover and if that's the case, he wants to go home.'

'But all of his meds ... and the outstanding results ...'

'Well ... that's what we wanted to discuss with you. Is there some way we can manage his symptoms *and* send him home?'

I paused. It wasn't something I had given much thought to. Jason was so reliant on medical care that the notion of him going home had never crossed my mind.

'It would be tricky ...'

'But possible?' Lisa asked.

'But probably possible,' I conceded. 'Also ... really complicated. He's on so many meds ...'

'Well, why don't we have a look at those?' said Mary. 'I've been going through the list and many of them have oral options. Aggie says if they're crushed, with a bit of banana, he can usually swallow most of them. We just need to find out from the pharmacist if crushing these meds is okay. The other thing to consider is putting them down his nasogastric tube.'

'Oh yeah,' I said. 'That reminds me. We can't send him home with an NG tube in place.'

'Why not?'

'Well, what if it comes out? Or something bad happens and it erodes through his stomach?'

'He can go to the nearby clinic and have one reinserted. As for the risks, he's well aware, but he's willing to accept them if it means he can go home.'

Every time I came up with a reason why Jason had to stay in hospital, Lisa and Mary gently and patiently provided a solution that would allow him to leave.

'It's just such a pity we don't have a paediatric hospice for him,' Mary sighed. 'He really would be an ideal candidate. There are no dedicated ones in the whole city. The local government keeps saying it wants to help out, but other projects are always prioritised.'

A paediatric hospice? This was simultaneously the best and worst thing I had ever heard of in my life. Who on earth would want to work there?

As we were wrapping things up, Lisa said, 'From a spiritual standpoint, Agnes would like an imam to come.'

'I ... had no idea she was Muslim,' I conceded. She had not worn any traditional Islamic garments or head covering and I had simply assumed she was Christian because of the Bible she carried with her.

'She's not, but Jason's father is and she would feel better if an imam saw him before he goes home. Jason says he feels closer to Muhammad than Jesus.'

'Okay! God, I didn't know that about his dad, I feel a bit silly ...'

'Nonsense!' Mary interjected. 'You run a busy ward with twenty-odd sick kids. You can't be expected to know every little detail about every one of them. That's why we're here.'

We went together to see Jason and I knelt down beside him and Agnes. 'Jason, I hear you want to go home, is that right?'

His head lolled over with difficulty and he whispered, 'Yes, Doctor. I miss my dog and my sister.'

'You understand that there won't be as much support if you go home, right? We won't be able to help you as quickly. We also probably won't be able to figure out what's wrong if you leave.'

'That's okay ...' he murmured and then smiled. Agnes nodded.

'I think we all know what's going on,' she said. 'If there was something you could do, you would have done it. Now it's in God's hands.'

When I got into my car later that afternoon, I decided to listen to something a little different on my drive home. My love of music had waxed and waned over the years and I had found myself in a bit of a rut. Indie rock, the staple of the noughties, found its star diminishing as the ingenuousness and sincerity of the decade were replaced with the anger and fear of the 2010s. Earnest white men strumming unselfconsciously on their guitars no longer had the same appeal it used to, but I hadn't found anything to replace it. I had cursorily glanced at a few year-end lists and saw the inclusion of a metal band called Deafheaven, with an album entitled *Sunbather*. Featuring a shockingly pink, distinctly un-metal cover to go with the un-metal album title, I was intrigued. Since my exposure to metal music in rehab, I was more open-minded and receptive to other music genres than before, but I hadn't really felt the need to return to metal. Nevertheless, this was a day for trying new things and I had always believed in considering art before rejecting it.

The album began mildly enough, with a single plaintive riff

climbing gently through a scale before being joined and harmonised by another. When the double bass and furious drums kicked in, I sensed I knew what was coming next, but what I wasn't prepared for was how, beneath the denseness of the guitars and the yelped vocals, there was a vulnerability. I couldn't decipher a single word of what was being sung, but I sensed the deep longing in the marrow of my bones. By the time I got to the final track on the album, I felt deeply, indescribably connected to the vicious distortion wringing through my head. Just as I thought the song was over and the album was ending with a pretty, if predictable, piano-driven outro, out of the blue, a final gut-rumbling riff thundered over me. I had just exited a petrol station to buy my energy drinks and a post-call coffee, and the sound knocked the air clean out of my lungs. There was only one thing left to do and that was swing into the ice-cream store on the way home and eat a cone while walking on the promenade. With Deafheaven in my head, and fudge-and-chocolate ice cream on my tongue, I watched the waves of the Atlantic crashing on the shore. I felt peace. It was a peace I wanted to extend to Jason. To find it, I had had to step outside my comfort zone. It was time to do that for him.

Over the next few days, we did what we could to get Jason home. Inessential medications were stopped or rationalised; a port IV line was inserted in his chest and the peripheral lines removed; and a clear and detailed plan was put together if he started deteriorating at home. Should he have to come back to hospital, simple instructions were made about limiting painful procedures that he didn't want. The PaedsPal team would visit him at his home in a few days to make sure everyone was coping.

Not every service was happy, however. I couldn't escape the mutters from some colleagues about how dangerous it was to be sending such a sick child home; how it was crazy to rely on his mother to provide specialised care and administer all his meds. A nurse would struggle, they murmured; his mother would be totally overwhelmed. They finished by remarking that we would likely never see or hear from Jason ever again and that his death would surely weigh on my conscience.

Yet Jason was more animated on the days before his discharge than I had ever seen him. His seizure frequency dropped; he smiled more; his mood visibly lifted. Even as it became clear that his underlying illness was progressing, the thought of living out his days where he wanted to be, surrounded by those he loved, energised him.

When Jason left, he was hugged by nearly every healthcare worker in the hospital. His smile could have powered the hospital for weeks. And even though moving his limbs had become excruciatingly painful, as he was wheeled out of the front gates, he turned and waved.

Jason died three weeks later, quietly at home, surrounded by those he loved and cuddling his dog. The PaedsPal team had visited him a few times to make sure everything was okay and to check that his mom was coping. He had required a brief admission to hospital when his seizures became unmanageable, but once we had adjusted his dose, we sent him home. His mother visited us shortly after Jason's death and brought us home-made biscuits. While the atmosphere was sombre, there was an undeniable spirit of celebration. Celebration for who Jason had been, not that he had been taken too soon.

She showed us photographs and some of Jason's schoolwork and laughed about his impish sense of humour. She told us that even at his young age, he had already developed an eye for the ladies; that his favourite cartoon was *South Park* (even though he was not supposed to watch it). What struck me was that by granting Jason a dignified, appropriate death, the PaedsPal team had allowed us all to focus on Jason's life, not on the manner of his passing. It didn't diminish the tragedy of a life lost too soon, but it granted us the gift of focusing on the aspects of Jason that had brought everyone so much joy. While no one explicitly commented on it, there was gratitude that his death hadn't overshadowed his life.

I contrasted this to many of the deaths I had witnessed as a paediatric registrar. Deaths where we had fought too hard, for too long, against the inevitable. While this may have assuaged the consciences of the doctors caring for a patient by allowing them to think we had 'tried everything', were we, in fact, doing our patients a disservice? Had we asked the patients and families of children with progressive, incurable conditions where they wanted to be for their final hours? Very few adults want to die in hospital surrounded by noisy machines, and I couldn't believe children would be any different. So why hadn't we asked? I had seen too many children spend their final hours surrounded by ventilators instead of family, with cold tubes and sharp needles in their bodies instead of a loving touch.

Every fibre of a paediatrician's being is geared towards saving life, almost regardless of the cost. But was that realistic? The truth is, for various reasons, not every child can survive to adulthood. Some have genetic or anatomical defects that severely restrict their health. Some are the victims of serious accidents or violence. Many have treatable illnesses but simply arrive at hospital too late. Regardless, it was drilled into us that 'children are not supposed to die. No parent should bury a child'. But it was becoming clearer and clearer to me that some children, tragically, *do* die, and we were doing a poor job in ensuring that their death was as pain- and symptom-free as possible. I had always thought there must be a better way and witnessing Jason's journey confirmed that for me.

PART 3: THE PRESCRIPTION

When the dust had settled, and I was debriefing with Mary and Lisa, Mary noted how passionate I had been about giving Jason a dignified send-off.

'You should consider doing a paediatric palliative care diploma,' she mentioned. 'It's a good thing our team happens to run one ...'

Driving home that afternoon, I felt I was at a crossroads. A palliative care diploma was never something I had really considered obtaining. It would be a year of intense work with regular assignments and lectures. Crucially, I was undecided about whether I wanted to go into general paediatrics or specialise further in something like infectious diseases. And yet. And yet a third path had suddenly materialised in front of me and I felt I was on the verge of something important. I had witnessed a better way and wanted to learn more. Nevertheless, I had a choice to make. For inspiration, I listened to *Sunbather* again (for the hundredth time). Suddenly, the parallels between palliative care and the music I was drinking in became inescapable. When I listened, I felt convinced I had stumbled on to some extraordinary secret known only to a select few. It was obvious to me that this was the best album I had heard in years. It was fresh and invigorating and shocking. Once you peeled away the screams and blast-beating drums, it was rich and complex and fascinating. It was also *way* off the usual path, and not something I ever thought I would enjoy. By taking a risk, an entire world had opened up to me. But this experience was not universal. I remembered how, at the beginning, I posted my thoughts on Facebook, urging everyone I knew to listen to *Sunbather*. After a few days of polite silence my friends replied that they found it completely unlistenable.

I didn't care. *Sunbather* didn't leave my car for eighteen months. The usual path was not for me. My music taste was about to change completely. And it wasn't the only thing.

Chapter 13
PAEDSPAL

By the time my four years as a paediatric registrar had ended, I was both exhausted and jobless. I had been a qualified doctor for nine years, but for the first time there was no clear path in front of me. I had been interested in super-specialising in paediatric infectious diseases but the only post in the province had been frozen and there were a host of other interested – and eminently qualified – candidates. Mostly, however, I just wanted to sleep.

I had calculated that the brutal ICU shift I had just completed was my 550th twenty-four-hour-plus call. I had spent the equivalent of a year and a half's worth of nights in various grimy, overloaded South African hospitals. I had missed more parties, birthdays, weddings, reunions and afternoon braais than I cared to remember. But what hurt the most was that while others were building shared memories with family and loved ones, my memories were of ill patients and lonely nights in dirty on-call rooms.

I had written yet another set of gruelling 'final' exams (every exam I wrote I swore would be the last and every few years more would come along), this time in paediatrics, spending my precious free time staring at notebooks and computer screens, memorising the minutiae of paediatric illnesses. I had written a thesis for my master's degree and begun renovations on a new house.

I was bone tired and needed a change of pace.

In my final few months as a registrar, a high-school student contacted me about the possibility of studying medicine. By any metric, this young woman was a superb candidate: straight As at school, a sterling public-service record and a variety of interesting and stimulating hobbies. Reading her CV made me grateful I was not having to compete with her for a spot at med school.

I had given the 'you should go into medicine' speech many times before – reeling off the reasons why being a doctor was a challenging, if fulfilling, career choice – when she asked me something that caught me off guard. She wondered: if I could go back in time to when I was in her shoes, would I still choose to study medicine? If, knowing what I knew now, would I put myself through it all?

My knee-jerk reaction was to say, 'Oh yes. Absolutely. Can't see myself happy doing anything else.' But the words caught in my throat. While I had no regrets about the choices I had made, was it true that this was the only career that would have made me happy? Was there perhaps another job out there that would have brought a similar amount of satisfaction, without the sacrifices I had made throughout my early twenties and thirties? I knew, of course, that many careers demanded a lot of studying and sacrifice, particularly at the beginning. But medicine, I felt, was the only career that demanded a portion of your very soul, and sometimes more. At its core, her question was both simple yet impossible to answer: was the cost of this path too high a price to pay? After a long silence, I mumbled something about pros and cons and quickly changed the subject. But the question remained in my mind.

I had seen too many colleagues walk away, watched so many dedicated and passionate people become bitter and cynical, ground down by a failing healthcare system that was propped up, in large part, by the big hearts of its doctors. For the very first time, I began questioning whether it had all been worth it. I needed something to spark my passion again. And that was when Mary from PaedsPal called.

I got to know Mary quite well the previous year when I completed my paediatric palliative care diploma. Inspired by the care I had seen given to the children during my training, and filled with a deep sense that for our very sick patients we were often – with the best of intentions – getting things horribly wrong, I decided to take the group up on its offer of completing additional training. Some of my supervisors thought I was wasting my time. Palliative care was not a recognised specialty in South Africa, they argued, and would not set me up for any viable future career paths. I would be better off doing original research, which would look great on my CV. These words were fair, but they never sat well with me. I felt there was something more beneath the solicitous advice – an undercurrent of confusion and exasperation. 'Palliative care' was morbid, the words whispered, and 'paediatric palliative care' even more so. Who would want to spend their days learning about critically ill or dying children? Palliative care was the service you called when you had *failed*. When medicine, with its wondrous machines, mysterious medicines and impenetrable lexicon, had broken down in the face of illness. To be in palliative care was to be confronted daily not only with the weakness of the human body, but the frailty of the scaffolding that held up medicine itself. Who would want to see *that* every day?

I had followed my gut and taken the class.

Perhaps unsurprisingly, I was the only male in a group of

sixteen women. Although I was a good student, I was by no means exceptional, and struggled at times with some of the intangible concepts promoted by our palliative care team. If medicine itself seemed over-rigid and reliant on protocol, often at the expense of kindness and warmth, palliative care sometimes felt like it went the other way with endless hours of discussion about every conceivable issue, even those we had no hope of fixing. I had come from an environment where I was expected to see thirty patients a day. Now I was thrust into a situation where we would often spend an hour or more on a single case. It took some adjusting as my natural inclination was to go as quickly as possible, lest I fall behind and never catch up again (burned into me from a thousand outpatient clinics). This was something I had to temper and recalibrate within myself. But I also felt that the urgency I brought was helpful in moving things along when the complexity of a patient's ailments threatened to bog us down indefinitely.

As a registrar, some of the feedback I regularly received was 'Sometimes not detail-orientated enough. Focuses on the large problems but occasionally misses the fine print'. This criticism had never overly bothered me. While I acknowledged the importance of being careful and thorough, I favoured the idea that the patient's overall well-being and subjective sense of health trumped minor abnormalities on a lab report. I also believed that the stereotypical paediatric obsession with minutiae came at a cost. In our efforts to fix every tiny issue, we would hang onto patients for too long when what they really needed was to be left alone. Perhaps even discharged.

Palliative care, with its 'big picture but also let's focus on every single issue', was like a well-fitting shoe with a piece of Lego in it – both comfortable and uncomfortable at the same time. It played to some of my strengths but highlighted many of my weaknesses. I also found myself at odds with some of the ideas promoted. One of those was medically assisted death. I had always believed that what mattered above all else was quality of life. Although there are metrics that measure this, it is largely subjective. Nevertheless, I was firm in my conviction that when an individual felt the pain and distress of a medical condition outweighed the joy life brought them, they should have the right to bring that life to a peaceful conclusion, on their own terms.

Many of the palliative care physicians believed that life was sacred and should never be prematurely shortened. This was often driven by an underlying religious faith (where only God should have the power to end life and for humans to adopt this sacred responsibility was, at best, hubristic, and, at worst, an outright deviation from God's plan for us). There was also concern that if we started to assist unwell people to die, we would be at the top of a slippery eugenic slope that ended in the removal of humans who were a burden on society. They argued that we had the tools and medications at our disposal to alleviate all but the most severe forms of suffering. Adequate palliative care, they continued, rendered the need for medically assisted death unnecessary.

I remember feeling conflicted. The programme I used to stay sober asked me to accept that there was something bigger than me that I needed to trust; that there was a plan for each of us. Yet here I was promoting the idea that humans, and not this higher power, should be the ultimate arbiters of life and death.

While it was never stated outright, there was an underlying subtext to much of the palliative work we did: to what extent is suffering part of the tapestry of life? And should it be accepted and managed or should we try to avoid it altogether? Those who thought suffering was an inextricable part of the human experience felt that assisting patients with dying deprived them of a key component of what made life precious. It was in suffering, they argued, that we truly experience the divine. They pointed to the fact that every major religion, from Christianity to Islam, uses deprivation to bring adherents closer to God. The most sacred tenet of Christianity, they went on, was that Jesus suffered on the cross for our salvation.

Those who thought suffering was an unpleasant by-product of life claimed that ending suffering was a mercy, that we didn't expect our pets to suffer, so why would we expect humans to? That suffering, *per se*, held no intrinsic benefits and should be avoided or mitigated if we had the means. While I fell into the latter camp, I was torn. My 'suffering' in rehab (while nowhere near what these kids were experiencing) had been pivotal in discovering something bigger than me. Week after week, I sat in Twelve-Step meetings that drummed home the idea that everything we had experienced had not been in vain; that our personal struggles – no matter how painful they had been at the time – carried deeper meaning. We came to believe that sadness and loss had led us to a spiritual awakening and put us in a position to be able to help others. But was this adequate explanation? Or simply retrospectively justifying pain and suffering? And could I have found my way to where I was without the need to suffer?

Among the PaedsPal group we never managed to change each other's minds, but it raised some interesting questions. While there was plenty written about what adults at the end of their lives attached meaning to, and the way they handled suffering, there was very little on children. What mattered to them? How did they view the end of their life? What else provided them with meaning?

A quick literature search yielded little. There were plenty of articles on what *adults* thought children found important, but precious little on the views of kids themselves. I decided I would try to explore this further, but before I could the diploma ended.

I had assumed our different beliefs ruled out any close collaborations between PaedsPal and myself, so when Mary offered me a temporary position to cover for Lisa who had gone on maternity leave, I couldn't help but express my surprise. When Mary heard my reservations, she laughed. 'If we only ever worked with people who shared our exact convictions the team would be very small indeed. The truth is that we need another paediatrician and you're one of the very few we would trust with our patients. What do you say?'

Once again, life had thrown me a curveball and I found myself joining Cape Town's first paediatric palliative care team, PaedsPal.

In the early days, I didn't know what I was doing. There was no palliative service offered to any of Cape Town's paediatric hospitals or wards, so we were in completely uncharted territory. We ran on a shoestring budget from a bunch of stakeholders, mostly private donors. We had a small office in Rondebosch, and a team consisting of a handful of physicians, a social worker, a nurse, a massage therapist, a receptionist and a whole lot of heart and goodwill.

When you are part of something new and fresh, something that feels *important*, there's a lot of nervous energy and excitement. But we also knew that from an outside perspective, our service was a tough sell. In a cash-strapped medical system, where every cent counts, convincing sceptical healthcare administrators to fork out on holistic care for complex and dying patients was a daily struggle. Whenever we made the pitch to hospital boards, quizzical eyebrows were raised, followed by grumblings of 'Shouldn't we spend the money trying to save them?' When we pointed out that not every child *could* be saved, that life had determined that some would have a short journey, all we heard was a clearing of throats, followed by nods to move onto the next item on the agenda.

When I started, our team only serviced the Red Cross Children's

Hospital. We knew from early on that there was a huge need beyond just one tertiary hospital for paediatric palliative care. Our team was small and very thinly stretched, but we quickly identified that many of the private hospitals in the Western Cape could be approached. There was also the promise that the funding from these hospitals, and the large medical aids that middle-class South Africans rely upon, could be used to bolster the meagre resources of PaedsPal. I decided to take the plunge and contact them.

The initial response was muted, to put it mildly. PaedsPal wrote a passionate missive to every CEO and administrator at these private hospitals, justifying why they should consider our services. We attached scientific papers clearly demonstrating the benefits of palliative services. We used stories from patients' families who had found our service helpful. The response was a stunning silence. When I followed up a week later, one lowly bureaucrat wrote back saying, 'Sorry, we already have those clown people who come sometimes to make the sick children laugh.'

We decided to try a different tack and sent the hospitals some data showing that palliative care *saved* money in the long run as happier, pain-free patients require less work from staff, fewer interventions and shorter stays in hospital. That hospitals looking out for their bottom lines should be even more interested in what we offered if money was the concern. Once again, we heard nothing.

In desperation, we contacted the physicians directly. This was slightly more effective, but confusion still reigned. When I did receive consult requests, it was often far too late in the patient's clinical course to make a meaningful difference. I was called in on a case to help a family with end-of-life care for a boy called Sam, who had been on a ventilator for over six months, with lungs that were beyond repair, and who was ineligible for a lung transplant. The decision had already been reached not to escalate care further, but the doctors wanted to slowly withdraw care as they felt it was causing ongoing harm, with no chance of recovery. I was brought in to try to 'sell' this idea to Sam's family; to make a stunningly difficult call more palatable.

I was angry at first. I didn't think it was my job to convince hesitant parents to consent to withdrawal of care. I felt palliative care should have been involved a lot earlier (a theme that would recur frequently as the months went on) and that we were being thrust into an unfair and complicated situation without care or due diligence. But after meeting with Sam's parents, my heart softened. Yes, the situation wasn't ideal, but there was still good we could achieve. I recalled what Chloe once said to me during my trauma internship at Baragwanath: 'You don't let a patient suffer because you're angry with a colleague.'

When it comes to their critically ill children, almost all parents would do anything for them. Anything at all. Most would stand in front of a bus, endure any suffering, give up any joy, forgo any luxury, if it meant their child would recover. They feel that anything less than an all-out attempt to find a cure would be a terrible failure as a parent; that they would only be able to sleep properly at night knowing that everything that could be tried had been tried. Many won't even entertain any other thoughts, as if contemplating anything except a total cure or recovery is a betrayal of their child and a black mark on their commitment to parenting.

But every medical intervention comes with a cost. That cost can be financial (a very real concern when medical aids dry up and refuse to provide more funds); it can be emotional (the longer a child remains in hospital the worse the emotional strain, not just on them, but on their parents as individuals, their marriage and other siblings); and it can be physical. It's the last one that really gives parents pause. When you explain that tubes down the throat, needles in the veins, side effects from the medications, ongoing surgical procedures, broken skin from lying flat all day, all cause pain, and that this pain is cumulative, parents really take notice.

There comes a point (that's different for everyone) where this cumulative emotional and physical pain – the 'burden of suffering' – becomes too heavy and outweighs any good you may be trying to achieve. When you phrase their child's experience like this – that it's a constant evaluation of cost and benefit, a delicate balancing act with multiple spinning plates, involving a variety of possible outcomes, rather than the overly simplistic dichotomy of 'cure or death' – then re-evaluations do occur. Because while parents want to do everything for their kids, they also hate seeing them suffer. Parents feel their children's suffering in the marrow of their bones. Often, however, the parents have never had a picture painted for them and they feel the pressure to keep going, whatever the cost. There is another way, however, and sometimes they just need to be shown that it is acceptable – and often kind – to embrace a path where *quality* of remaining life, not *quantity*, is the goal.

I tried, gently, to explain the situation in full to Sam's parents and family. What amazed me from very early on was that there was already an understanding fully present inside them; they just needed a trusted professional to allow them to express it. They *knew* he was suffering. They *knew* the burden was too much to bear. But no one had ever given them permission to explore a path that didn't involve forging on for a cure at all costs.

We sat for hours. We discussed options. We discussed possible outcomes. We discussed best possible and worst possible scenarios. We cried. Everyone cried. After the first night, nothing was settled, but the door to another path had been opened.

Over the coming days, I went backwards and forwards with Sam's parents. Sometimes we disagreed. Sometimes we had to go over topics again and again. After examining Sam, I was able to make some minor, but significant adjustments to his medications, which provided him with immediate relief. The change in his overall demeanour was apparent to his family and this helped to build trust. I was no longer 'The Death Doctor' and instead, I was becoming 'The Pain Relief Doctor'. It wasn't a perfect description of me (or palliative care, which is more holistic than that), but it was certainly preferable, and so I ran with it.

Every evening, I would feed back to Mary, who would advise me on possibilities or options I hadn't considered. I, in turn, would have discussions with Sam's medical team about how the process was going. There was initial frustration at how long it was taking. Sam's suffering was evident to all his healthcare professionals, but because no palliative conversations had ever taken place with his family, there was a gulf between where his doctors and parents were in the process. Bridging this gap would take time, I explained.

Throughout the journey, I felt Sam and his pain wherever I went. And he was just one of several palliative patients I was seeing at the time.

There is no weight as heavy as a child's pain and everyone involved in their care carries it. I thought about Sam when I was at the grocery store. I worried about him while I tried to sleep at night. His pain and groans would accompany me on my evening runs. I felt tired most of the day and my shoulders constantly ached. The only time I didn't think about him, and my other palliative patients, was when I lost myself in the furious blasts of Norwegian black metal, or the sinuous, chaotic chords of dissonant death metal. In the furious oblivion, I rediscovered what I had found in rehab: the brutal music's ability to provide an outlet for rage and sadness, to distract from the unthinkable and, ultimately, to soothe. By now, I had discovered how massive the genre was and I could discern between the fury of black metal, the heaviness of death metal and the density of doom metal.

I spoke to a rabbi online who frequented one of the metal sites I liked to visit for recommendations, and when I expressed surprise that a rabbi was a metalhead, he expressed surprise that a paediatrician was one, too. I had never thought of myself as a 'metalhead' before, but the truth was, I was listening to metal more than any other type of music. I asked the rabbi what a religious man took from it. His response was 'All music is a conversation with God. Sometimes, it's gentle and soothing. Metal is the furious spit in the face. Don't worry: God can take it.' I stopped trying to analyse why I loved the music and began to simply enjoy it on its own terms. Eventually I was listening to it whenever I had a spare moment, especially at night. To the amazement of my friends and family, I'd listen to extremely loud heavy metal music just before bed to help me sleep.

To supplement my relatively meagre income from PaedsPal (no private hospital had paid me yet, and our funds were paper thin), I was also doing general paediatric locums at a private clinic in Tygerberg. I was standing in for a kindly, elderly community paediatrician whenever he went to Poland to visit his family.

I was good at the work and the communication skills I had learned during the PaedsPal diploma were playing a major role in my chats to parents and kids. But there was a darker side, too.

I had to try to separate my palliative patients from the ones being brought to me by worried parents in the wealthier suburbs of Cape Town and Stellenbosch. It wasn't easy. The contrast between the critically ill – often dying – kids I saw regularly as a palliative physician, and the temporarily sick – but generally fine – kids I saw in private care was stark. Sometimes they bled into each other. One morning a child came in with a viral throat infection. She was clearly distressed, but not more so than thousands of children I had seen just like her who needed some mild analgesia and a good nap. In my overly concerned way, I ended up creating a multi-layered pain guideline, with provisos and contingency plans should her pain not improve.

'Doctor. It's just her tonsils. This has happened a few times before and she was okay with some antibiotics and Panado. All this what-what planning is freaking us out.'

I ditched the plan. But for the rest of the day, I couldn't get the thought out of my head that her throat might close completely, that she might die, that it would all be my fault. I phoned her family later that day to check she was okay. She had slept peacefully all afternoon but I was a quivering wreck on the way to my car.

After a week or so, we had a breakthrough with Sam's family. His parents had given it a lot of thought and decided they didn't want him to suffer any further. Over the weekend, his mother had explained to him what was going on and she had felt him squeeze her hand. This, to her, was a sign that he agreed that it was time to stop.

I ran over the plan with his family. With medications and other means we were going to make sure he was comfortable and pain-free. We weren't going to give him anything to hasten his death (which we were prohibited from doing anyway), but we were going to stop the exceptional measures that were keeping him alive. In other words, we were going to allow nature to take its inevitable course. We had plans for what would happen if he went quickly, and plans for what we would do if he decided to stay with us for a while. At all times, Sam's well-being remained foremost in our minds.

On the evening we withdrew care, Sam's entire extended family visited him in the ICU. Some came individually, others in groups. Young cousins, toddler cousins and old, wizened grandparents alike paid their respects and said goodbye. He was hugged and kissed and showered with love. Flowers and his favourite toys adorned his bed. Everybody commented how Sam had forever changed their lives with his cheeky smile and kind heart. Tears flowed for a life so tragically cut short. It was strange for me to hear how Sam was before he became sick because I had never had the chance to have a proper conversation with him. I had only ever known the critically ill boy on a ventilator in the ICU.

I think I would have enjoyed getting to know Sam. There was an internal ache because I had to navigate both participating in the grief while being apart from it. I had to be both mourner and physician at the same time. The tears being shed were so genuine, how could I add mine when I barely knew him? They flowed anyway and I wondered if I was a fraud.

When we were ready, we removed the endotracheal tube, stopped the artificial ventilation and put him onto an oxygen mask. I will never know for sure, but I think I detected a hint of a smile. There was a huge exhalation, a squeeze of his mother's hand, and then he was gone.

While his family mourned, I completed paperwork.

That afternoon, I had to rush off to see a full general paediatric clinic.

Chapter 14
WHAT MAKES YOU HAPPY?

After Sam, I was convinced I could make a real difference – that there was a serious need for paediatric palliative care in Cape Town. But the next few patients I saw went very differently. In some cases, the parents were simply not ready to even discuss the option of palliative care. In one case I was ushered into a huge conference room in a hospital and seated at one end of a long table, with the parents of a young boy seated at the other. The distance between us was completely unbridgeable, and when I tried to move closer to try to establish a human connection, his mother visibly recoiled and couldn't end the meeting fast enough. I heard later that she 'appreciated' my time but felt I had been 'too aggressive' in pushing my 'palliative agenda'.

In another case, when I broached the topic of possible end-of-life care, and the need to plan for it, a little girl's father became angry, insisting that he had googled 'palliative care' and knew that we were preparing for death. In his eyes, death was simply not an option, and he felt we had been brought in to 'trick him' into accepting it. His voice quavered and rose in such fury that I thought at one stage he was getting ready to punch me.

These encounters left me deflated and demoralised. Was I the problem? Was I somehow misrepresenting my field? Was I unintentionally antagonising grieving parents? Coming in too hot with discussions about death and suffering? Being too pushy? Not listening enough?

One of the most frustrating parts was not having anyone to talk to about any of it. Who could I broach about these issues? Mary was always sympathetic but was incredibly busy with her own patients, the palliative care diploma, and trying to keep PaedsPal afloat. My wife was busy with her own training and we barely saw each other. I had gradually drifted away from AA and NA meetings and no longer had a sponsor. After years of therapy around my time in rehab, I felt 'analysed out' and resisted seeing a psychologist. I was lonely and struggling, trying to lead a normal existence while dealing with the most abnormal pain and anguish in my palliative patients every day.

One day I was talking to a palliative inpatient about her feeding issues. She was seven years old and the nausea from her medications was intolerable. Keeping her fed and hydrated was proving to be a real challenge. Yet she seemed upbeat. I was feeling beaten down and heavy by my failures and my curiosity eventually got the better of me.

'Evangeline, there's so much going on and you're so sick yet you look happy. What's your secret? We adults would like to know.' I was only half joking.

'My dog! Rufus!'

'What about him?'

'The hospital let him visit me today.'

I remembered how close she was to the golden retriever her parents had bought for her when it seemed like she was in remission.

I also thought way back to fourth year, and how Mr Peterson, with the terrible bowel disease, had only improved when he knew his dog was being cared for. Although animals are generally not allowed in hospitals, we had applied to the hospital administrators for special permission for Rufus to visit. I assumed they would say no, but someone higher up had taken pity and signed off on it. I was sad I hadn't been informed and had missed the happy reunion, but this was part of a general pattern I was noticing. For whatever reason, palliative care physicians often weren't taken as seriously as some of our counterparts.

After being cleansed and shampooed to within an inch of his life, Rufus was given permission to visit his favourite human. Even though he had been whisked away after only a few minutes of cuddles and petting, the effect on Evangeline was profound. She was sitting up in her bed and colouring in, something she hadn't had the energy to do for days. There was a warm pinkness to her cheeks and she was humming a nursery rhyme to herself. For the first time in a long time, there was a feeling of life emanating from her weak body. I scooted a little closer.

'Evangeline. *Why* does Rufus make you so happy?'

She looked up and gave me a puzzled look. 'Duh. He's a dog! We all love our dogs! That was a silly question.' Then she resumed her colouring. Although she was clearly done with me, I felt I had stumbled onto something either extremely banal or profoundly important. Maybe both. I decided to press her a little more.

'What else makes you happy? You know ... when you're in hospital?'

She gave a loud sigh, irritated at the interruption, but nevertheless brought her pencil to her mouth while she pondered the question.

After a few seconds, she shrugged. 'I like ... Wonder Woman!

She's brave and pretty.' She nodded vigorously, as if confirming this excellent opinion. 'I want to be like her. And ... and I like ... when my mummy reads to me.'

'Is that all?' I was scrounging around in my backpack for a notebook to write this stuff down.

'That's all!' she said cheerily, before resuming her colouring in. I knew there was more to it than that but I didn't want to disturb her any further. I made a mental note to ask every patient I encountered over the next few weeks about the things that made them happy. The stuff that brought them joy and meaning; that reduced the pain and restored life. I wasn't wholly prepared for the response.

Over the course of the following weeks, I heard a lot about Superman. And Batman. And Spiderman. And Iron Man. And The Incredible Hulk. I always knew kids loved superheroes, but until I really explored the topic, I had no idea how inspirational they were to those in distress. The kids I spoke to drew strength from the worlds of Marvel and DC. They analogised their illnesses to the common superhero trope of being different to everyone and yet the same. Of sticking out when you want to fit in. Of following the hard path even when you didn't want to. Of bravery even when hope seems lost.

It was interesting that the medium of the story affected the children in very different ways. While they all enjoyed the movies and TV shows, it was comic books and graphic novels that truly enchanted them. One day I took in a giant graphic novel of Marvel stories for a young boy who was a fan of the character Thor. When he and his mother saw the size of the book, there was an awkward pause.

'We're grateful for the gift, Doctor. But he doesn't read so good and the pain means he struggles to concentrate. Maybe when he's a bit better?' His mother sounded embarrassed. I said that was fair, but I left it by his bedside just in case. After I had examined him and was on my way out, I turned around and said, 'Ever wondered who would win if Thor and Hulk battled it out?'

'Thor,' he answered without looking up or missing a beat.

'Are you sure?'

He paused.

'Because they battle each other in chapter four. It's *epic*. Maybe read it and put your theory to the test?'

The next day when I arrived, he was fast asleep. The giant book was resting on his belly, which was softly rising and falling with each quiet breath. His mother told me that once he had started reading the novel, he had become so engrossed that tearing him away proved nearly impossible. Eventually, he had closed his eyes just after 10pm and had his best night's sleep in weeks. She said that the comic had grabbed his attention in a completely different way to the TV shows. He had felt connected to the object he was holding, invested in a way that consumed his imagination and provided joy that distracted him from the pain in his bones. When he woke up, the first thing he asked was if there were more books available to read. I smiled.

It wasn't just comics. The kids were passionate about stories in general. Nothing made them happier than being read to by a loved one. The sense of being the sole focus of the reading parent; the strands of proximity that the spoken words tied together invisibly; the anticipation of what would come next, even when a story had been shared a hundred times before. The absolute peace and wonder never diminished. I watched as the words gently washed over the children, and they drifted into a sleep peopled by pirates and unicorns and talking sharks and fairies. They all considered this time priceless.

They all loved the physical activities many of their healthy friends took for granted. From running on grass, to building sandcastles on the shore and swimming in the sea, they treasured using their bodies in the outdoors. Incredibly, there was rarely any jealousy about healthy peers for whom these activities were totally normal, just a fond reminiscence of times gone by, and a hope they would be able to feel the sand beneath their toes sometime soon.

When it was safe, organising events outside the hospital could be life-changing for these kids. One weekend the PaedsPal team managed to take two chronically ill children to the Two Oceans Aquarium. The logistics were as complex as they were daunting, as the team had to transport wheelchairs, accommodate ventilators, keep essential medication nearby and have healthcare workers available in the event of an emergency. PaedsPal did this with a smile and for free. The two kids couldn't stop talking about it for days afterwards. It was like they had won the lottery, not done something most children do so regularly that they take it for granted. A simple change of scenery, being in nature, getting out of the fluorescent harshness of the hospital, being able to 'move' for just a little while. The meaning and joy the kids squeezed from every second were unquantifiable.

On days when such a huge undertaking was not possible, just getting out onto the lawn and experiencing some sunshine had a huge rejuvenating effect on the children. Cool grass between our toes, the soil on our heels, the dappled shade of a tree, all provide spiritual sustenance. We underestimate how much we lose when we can't even go outside. When I asked one of the girls what she would love to do next, more than anything in the world, she answered, 'Go to the beach and build a sandcastle.'

Humour was something that caused the pain to melt away. I quickly discovered that there is no Dad joke too Dad-jokey for kids. ('What's big, grey, weighs a thousand kilos and wears slippers?

Cinderelephant!') I discovered that kids enjoy telling jokes as much as they enjoy hearing them, and once it had been established that I enjoyed both, it was common when kids saw me walk through the door to yell, 'I've got one! What's brown and sticky?' (A stick) or 'What did the vet say to the cat?' (How are you feline?)

In addition, kids love physical and slapstick comedy. Farts, funny noises, weird faces and unfortunate accidents are all a constant source of delight. Even the most stoic child will collapse in a heap of giggles when they witness an adult do something silly. It is as if humour and laughter are competitors at pain receptor sites; the more someone is laughing and enjoying themselves, the less physical pain they feel. Or perhaps they do feel it, but it is simply lessened. Children who are in pain feel sad and sadness worsens the pain. Breaking this vicious cycle is often very difficult, but few things are as effective as mirth. And no silliness is too silly for children (until they become teenagers and then nothing an adult does intentionally is funny any more). Much of what we said and discussed was incredibly serious, yet these moments of levity scattered throughout the day were priceless.

Authenticity was craved, especially by the older kids and teens. I once struggled to get through to a teenage boy who had been in hospital for weeks with a terrible tumour, complicated by one set of bad news after the other. When I tried to speak to him, he put his headphones on and began blaring his music. I was disheartened until one day I realised that he was listening to metal, more precisely (and I swear this is true) the furious tones of Emperor. I was immediately taken back to Tabankulu when I was first exposed to metal by my roommate, and more specifically to the band Emperor. The boy was listening to the same album that had barged its way into my eardrums fifteen years before when I was a patient. I was immediately transported back, in the way only music can do, to a time when I was angry, desperate and vulnerable. I was reminded of how I felt and what ultimately pulled me though.

Was it chance? Or something bigger? I'll never know. But this time I knew a lot more about what I was hearing. I was ready.

Black metal was conceived in the eighties but popularised in the nineties by a group of misanthropic Norwegian bands. Emperor was one of them. The sound is characterised by tremolo guitars, rapid-fire blast beats and furious, unmelodic rasps. There's the frequently amateurish production (sometimes described as 'raw', which is a charitable way of saying it often sounds like it was recorded inside a trash can); the black-and-white corpse paint band members wear to appear evil and demonic, and finally, the chaotic music itself. Those Norwegian bands took the existing template of a burgeoning new sound, made it even more oppressive, and birthed an entirely new aesthetic altogether (denoted as the 'Second Wave of Black Metal'). Black metal has morphed tremendously since then. These days, bands have swapped the corpse paint for faded jeans and T-shirts, and much of the early stuff now seems a bit hokey and silly. But for aficionados there is something alluring about the harsh atmosphere of the Norwegian progenitors. In the eyes of the hardened metalhead, liking these bands is to be 'kvlt' – a 'true fan' not a 'hipster metal tourist'.

To non-metalheads this brand of music is completely and utterly unlistenable. Everything about it is designed not just to put off casual music geeks, but to actively repel them. For fans of the sub-genre, however, Emperor are to black metal what The Beatles are to rock 'n roll.

By playing this music while I was supposed to be talking to the boy, he was not so subtly telling me to fuck off. He figured that if his silence didn't scare me away, his scary taste in music would.

Unfortunately for him, I was in the one per cent of people who love black metal.

The next day, I dusted off my black Emperor T-shirt in my closet and took it to the hospital. Before entering his room, I put it on. A black metal logo is often like a doctor's handwriting, completely impenetrable unless you're familiar with it. He took one look at my shirt, his eyes widened, and then narrowed as disbelief shifted to suspicion. He knew there was a shared, private language, but he was suspicious.

'Where did you get that shirt?'

'In Norway. Oslo, to be precise. I found it at a store there. Why?'

'You like Emperor?'

'Hell yeah, I like Emperor! *In the Nightside Eclipse* is one of the best black metal albums of all time.'

'I think you mean *Anthems to the Welkin at Dusk*.'

I gently took his arm to feel his pulse. It was the first time he had let me touch him.

'*Anthems* is a great album, to be sure. But it lacks the menace of *Eclipse*. And there are no songs that touch "I am the Black Wizards", I'm afraid,' I said.

'How can you even say that ...' By now I was palpating his abdomen, '... have you never heard "With Strength I Burn"?' he objected.

'A banger, sure. But *Eclipse* was the first Emperor album I heard, and you love your first, you know?' My hands had shifted to the large ulcer on his leg. He hadn't let anyone examine it before. He flinched and raised his guard again.

'Any other bands you like? Anyone can Google stuff these days.'

'Well, we just sticking to black metal? Or can I go broader? How about death metal? Doom? Thrash? If we're talking something a bit more modern, I'm really digging the latest Khemmis – it's called

Hunted. If you're into doom with chonky riffs, give it a bash. In fact ...' My hands had gone back to his leg again and this time he stayed still. '... if you like, I can bring you some stuff to try tomorrow. And I'd love it if you could make some recommendations for me. I'm always on the lookout.'

'How heavy do you like it? The stuff I like isn't for the faint-hearted.'

'Nothing you've got is heavier than the album in my car at the moment. It's black-hole heavy and face-meltingly fast. You won't be able to top it.'

He smiled. 'Challenge accepted.'

Over the next few days, we exchanged music. We discussed metal bands no one in the room had heard of. Crucially, he let me examine him and discuss his health. When I made some recommendations he didn't like, he rolled his eyes and said, 'Fiiiiiiiiinnnneee. But only because you're not a total dork like everyone else here.' He gestured vaguely around him. I knew by this stage that he was all bark and no bite and that he got on extremely well with Nomzamo, one of his nurses. But I was touched anyway. His dad pulled me aside as I left his room one day and drew me into a corner.

'Do you really like these awful metal bands? Or do you deserve an Oscar?'

I laughed. 'I get this a *lot*. It's not an act. I like the music.'

'Well ... thank God someone does because you're the only doctor he's opened up to. All because you both like bands called Cattle Decapitation and SepticFlesh'. He shook his head. 'I'll never understand. But thank you for having terrible taste in music.'

It wasn't the first time I had heard that line. I smiled at the way the universe sometimes worked.

Chapter 15
THE HEALING PROPERTIES OF ICE CREAM

As MONTHS PASSED AND I ASKED MORE QUESTIONS, MORE THEMES EMERGED. I realised that some answers took longer because the kids needed a piece of me before they were willing to share a piece of themselves. The teenage metalhead only opened up when he knew I was also a metalhead. The kids who liked superheroes wanted to see I was a fan first before telling me who their favourite one was. Initially, this was difficult because we had been taught not to share too much of ourselves with patients, lest we lose objectivity. They are patients, not friends, we were told. You need to maintain professional boundaries. There was also the notion that the patient was the centre of the discussion, not the doctor. By talking about yourself you were framing their illness through your lens and not respecting theirs. None of this was bad advice, but I soon understood that patients want to be treated by human beings not automatons. This wasn't a groundbreaking discovery (like all medical students, I had watched *Patch Adams* many times and, while I found the movie cloying and melodramatic, I agreed with its underlying message), but in an era of higher rates of litigiousness, and with Facebook blurring the lines between public and private, very few physicians were willing to share anything of themselves with their patients. When I opened up just a tiny fraction, the kids responded accordingly. They let me continue to find out what made them happy.

Nothing was more important than family. The memories that lingered with the greatest force in the kids' minds were those of happy times with their parents, siblings, cousins, uncles, aunts and grandparents. Holidays, meals out, movies, or just simple picnics ... there was simply no substitute for quality family time. There was an especially cruel irony in this because there is no greater stressor on a family unit than one of the kids being unwell in hospital. Many relationships simply don't survive the planet-dense weight of a suffering or dying child, and either snap suddenly, or gradually crumble. It is a terrible cruelty that the element many children draw on for strength is the same element often being snuffed out by their illness. The kids felt this acutely. They were, almost without exception, intensely worried about their parents and siblings. Incredibly, many even worried about the effect their death would have on their loved ones, and how those loved ones would cope moving forward. A little boy, near the end of his life, told me that he was worried that his mum would be 'too sad' when he was gone, but that he would 'always be there' looking over her. Many seemed certain there would be a reunion sometime in the future, which they were looking forward to. They felt, deep down, that this state was temporary. They were certain that, even in death, better days lay ahead.

Kindness was something the kids valued almost above any other trait. Importantly, while they valued *words* of kindness, these only mattered if backed by *acts* of kindness. Meaningless platitudes

('You're so brave', in particular, irritated many of them because it's not how they saw themselves), insincere positivity ('It's all going to be okay!' when they knew something was very wrong), and fake promises ('I won't let anything bad happen to you!') were all counterproductive. Children are very good at seeing through bullshit, especially from adults they know and trust. When kindness was manifested through sincere actions (a nurse being especially gentle while changing an IV dressing, friends sharing their toys, a family member holding them or taking extra time to be with them), it carried enormous power. Chronically ill children live and breathe Maya Angelou's famous words, 'At the end of the day, people won't remember what you said or did, they will remember how you made them feel.' You don't have to mislead a child to make them feel happy, you just have to make them feel loved and special.

FaceTime with siblings, letters from classmates, an unexpected visitor ... these all rated far higher than the cool new PlayStation game or funky gadget. There was, however, no kindness more valued than simply having one or both caregivers *present*. Not necessarily doing anything, just present in the moment.

Nothing takes people *away* from the moment quite like electronics. People (and I am guilty of this) disappear into their screens. For many parents, this was probably a relief – a few moments when they didn't have to focus on the enormity of their stress and could abandon themselves into other people's lives and struggles. But when viewed over prolonged periods, they sapped the attention of loved ones to such an extent that they appeared, at times, like disinterested robots.

Having caregivers both physically and emotionally present wasn't always possible, especially for kids who had been in hospital for a long time, but it was valued beyond anything else. Put simply,

PART 3: THE PRESCRIPTION

the most valued commodity wasn't time but *meaningful* time focused on the present.

As I was writing all of the kids' responses down, I noticed something interesting. None of the kids (even the older ones) had said anything about social media. There was no mention of wanting more friends, or likes, or followers; no lamentations about not spending more time looking at the shenanigans of celebrities. Given how often I see kids scrolling through TikTok, Instagram or Facebook, this surprised me. I decided to categorically ask some of them about this. Did seeing other kids leading 'normal' lives perhaps make them sad? Were they too tired and weakened to keep up with the never-ending flow of information? Did their suffering render the minor day-to-day bumps and bruises of life that others were caught up in seem silly? The responses were surprising. One young girl commented, 'If I post anything, I just get a million responses with hearts and rainbows and people telling me how inspirational I am, or whatever. And I'm like, "But what about the actual thing I posted!? Did none of you read it?" It's, like, on social media, they can't see beyond my illness ...'

Another young boy noted, 'Social media isn't real. It's people being artificially controversial, or happy, or whatever. And I just don't have time for anything that's not real.'

One teenager told me, 'I kinda wished I hadn't worried so much about stupid social media. No one cares. It's not real. It's cool sometimes to see what my friends are up to ... but beyond that ...' She shrugged.

I asked many of them what else they thought had been a waste of time and energy. An insightful response I got from a young girl captured it all. She said, 'I wish I hadn't worried so much about what other people thought of me. Especially people who didn't matter.

I was so embarrassed about the baldness and the weight, but my real friends didn't care. Some people will just always be mean. Adults pretended that nothing was different, which was lame, but my friends just carried on like it was no big deal. Which was cool. Pretending is dumb.'

The kids also noted that many of the things they were worried about – scars, ports, stitches – were often the very things other people noticed last. Mostly, they just wanted to be treated like everyone else and they found grand and expansive gestures acknowledging their frailties to be unnecessary at best and embarrassing and distracting at worst.

Ice cream. Every single kid loved it. The joy of being handed a cone scooped with different colours of creamy goodness, the anticipation of that first lick, the curiosity of how the exciting new flavour would taste, the tingliness of the cream and sugar on the tongue and lips, the strategy of how best to mould the icy tower with their tongues, the satisfied crunch of the first bite into the cone ... Every moment was a delightful one to savour. Beyond the sugar and cream, there was relief at the soothing of mouths rendered raw by chemotherapy, of lips chapped by dry hospital ventilation, of tummies shrunken by endless bland hospital food.

Ice cream was a treat, a joy, a guilty pleasure. Best of all, it could be shared. I lost count of how many times a child and parent would lick their ice cream, look at each other, share a silent moment of joyful acknowledgement and then collapse into giggles. There is something uniquely special about ice cream. Every kid (and adult) agreed.

After a few weeks, I gathered up all the notes I had scribbled. I then tried to organise them in a coherent manner. It was heartbreaking work coming across a fragment of an idea from a patient who I realised had since passed on. The wisdom of what I was holding felt even more profound.

There was nothing here that hadn't been said or philosophised before, but never had I seen innocence and wisdom laid out so clearly and cleanly. I also realised that it was not an accident; right *now* was the time for me to document this. Everything that had happened had led me to the point where I was clinically experienced enough, emotionally secure enough, and scarred and healed enough, that the children trusted me. I was by no means perfect, but kids don't demand perfection, just a sign that you're trying your best and have their interests at heart. I also realised this was a message meant to be shared.

I thought back to the privileged but damaged boy who found himself addicted to alcohol, cast out from medical school, who had to find the spiritual strength, the internal honesty and reliance on others to claw his way back. I did a quick calculation and determined that I had been sober for well over a decade. For an addict or alcoholic, every day sober is a miracle. I had allowed time to dampen the enormity of that achievement but it was crucial. Without sobriety, nothing followed. I still say the Serenity Prayer whenever I'm feeling overwhelmed. I do not know who, or what, God is (or if He/She even exists). But I know, at my lowest ebb, when I reached out, something reached back. That's enough.

I had recently tried to reconnect with some of my friends from rehab. Catching up was as disheartening as it was sobering. Joe – the 'Captain Recovery' from my early days – had recently died. Despite multiple attempts at getting better, he was never able to string together a significant stretch of sobriety. He had passed away of heart failure, induced by alcohol damage, a few months before. It was tragic how many lives this terrible illness took. I calculated that of the people I had been in rehab with, twelve had died directly as a result of their addiction. Those were only the ones I knew of; the number was likely higher. Many others were either in jail or in mental-health facilities. Chad, the cynical seventeen-year-old, had been admitted for intractable depression and drug abuse. Not all tales were depressing, however. Mike, the Brit who had shown me mercy and kindness at Tabankulu, had found sobriety, returned to the UK, and opened a string of successful rehabs. Many of my co-patients had become counsellors or psychologists and were using their skills to help others. The primary rehab I went to still stands and still provides a haven for people to get better. It's just a tragedy that many who desperately need this resource are unable to access it for financial reasons.

Jim, the owner of Tabankulu, had tragically suffered a heart attack and passed away a few years earlier. The beating heart of Tabankulu stopped with his and it closed shortly thereafter. I was saddened by the news because it was such a unique place. It was where, between the cold and rain and chopping of wood and exposure to metal music, I had found recovery and healing. The extended nature of the programme, which initially made me feel so disheartened, is what helped me and so many others ultimately get better. I'm not aware of any similar facilities in Cape Town.

I cast my mind back to the intern who stumbled into Chris Hani Baragwanath, and how that intern was just a young, damaged man whose skin needed to harden, but who perhaps allowed part of his soul to callous in the process. I laughed at the dramas that unfolded, the larger-than-life personalities I had encountered, the long nights and even longer post-call days. In many ways it had broken me down to build me back up, but the cost was steep.

Mandy was still in the US working for a pharmaceutical company.

She had texted intermittently in the first few years, but we had drifted apart. Kobus was working as a GP in Limpopo and is a proud husband and father. He recently ran his tenth Comrades marathon and still smokes the odd cigarette.

Phelo went into obstetrics and gynaecology and is now a consultant working in Gauteng. He remains politically active to this day. Anwar and Angela both became internal medicine consultants and practise in Gauteng and Durban respectively.

Chloe took some time off from her registrar time after the separation from Dr Simpson, but came back a few months later and completed it, winning the academic medal for her year. She met a new guy and followed him back to Mauritius, where she now works.

Prof Waters ultimately retired but is still amassing a book of collective nouns. The marijuana field (I'm told) lives on.

The most important legacy of Bara is that it didn't break me. It taught me to hang in when times got tough, to rely on others when I needed to, and to resist the urge to treat people as numbers or problems. After Bara, some people walk away. I just took a different path. A more winding one, a more complicated one, a more unusual one. It had led me here, to a place of wisdom and understanding. Now I just needed to share it.

Reflections on Going Viral

D*UDE! YOU'RE EVERYWHERE!*
I stared at the text on my phone, confused. It was from a close friend of mine living in London.

What do you mean? I hurriedly texted back. I was out with friends and didn't want to appear rude.

That thread on Twitter – It's all over the news! Everyone's talking about it!

At that moment, my phone started to vibrate. It didn't stop for the next two hours. Texts and WhatsApps from family and friends asking if I was the author of a thread that was rapidly circling the globe; journalists trying to get in touch; members of the public reaching out; Twitter notifications that began as a river, but one that started to rapidly flood and soon quickly burst its banks. The more I tried to keep up the further I was falling behind. And then, quite suddenly, with more than fifty per cent of its battery remaining, my phone decided it had had enough and shut down. I exhaled. What the hell had just happened?

After collating all the kids' thoughts I had collected over the past few months, I had decided earlier that day, rather randomly, to post them on the app formerly known as Twitter. At the time I had a modest following (around 2 000 followers), and most of my tweets received around ten 'likes' and two or three 'retweets'. During my lunch break, I quickly composed a thread summarising what I had found. It went as follows:

🐦 **Alastair McAlpine**, MD @AlastairMcA30, 1 Feb. 2018

For an assignment, I asked some of my terminal paediatric palliative care patients what they had enjoyed in life, and what gave it meaning. Kids can be so wise, y'know. Here are some of the responses.
(Thread)

First:
NONE said they wished they'd watched more TV.
NONE said they should've spent more time on Facebook.
NONE said they enjoyed fighting with others.
NONE enjoyed hospital.
/1

MANY mentioned their pets:
'I love Rufus, his funny bark makes me laugh.'
'I love when Ginny snuggles up to me at night and purrs.'
'I was happiest riding Jake on the beach.'
/2

MANY mentioned their parents, often expressing worry or concern:
'Hope Mum will be okay. She seems sad.'
'Dad mustn't worry. He'll see me again soon.'
'God will take care of my mum and dad when I'm gone.'
/3

ALL of them loved ice cream.
/4

ALL of them loved books or being told stories, especially by their parents:
'Harry Potter made me feel brave.'
'I love stories in space!'
'I want to be a great detective like Sherlock Holmes when I'm better!'
Folks, read to your kids! They love it.
/5

MANY wished they had spent less time worrying about what others thought of them and valued people who just treated them 'normally':
'My real friends didn't care when my hair fell out.'
'Jane came to visit after the surgery and didn't even notice the scar!'
/6

MANY of them loved swimming, and the beach:
'I made big sandcastles!'
'Being in the sea with the waves was so exciting! My eyes didn't even hurt!'
/7

Almost ALL of them valued kindness above most other virtues:
'My granny is so kind to me. She always makes me smile.'
'Jonny gave me half his sandwich when I didn't eat mine. That was nice.'
'I like it when that kind nurse is here. She's gentle. And it hurts less.'
/8

PRESCRIPTION: ICE CREAM

Almost ALL of them loved people who made them laugh:
'That magician is so silly! His pants fell down and I couldn't stop laughing!'
'My daddy pulls funny faces, which I just love!'
'The boy in the next bed farted! Hahaha!'
Laughter relieves pain.
/9

Kids love their toys, and their superheroes:
'My Princess Sophia doll is my favourite!'
'I love Batman!' (All the boys love Batman.)
'I like cuddling my teddy.'
/10

Finally, they ALL valued time with their family. Nothing was more important.
'Mum and dad are the best!'
'My sister always hugs me tight.'
'No one loves me like mummy loves me!'
/11

Take-home message:
Be kind. Read more books. Spend time with your family. Crack jokes. Go to the beach. Hug your dog. Tell that special person you love them.
These are the things these kids wished they could've done more. The rest is details.
Oh ... and eat ice cream.
/End

I had pushed 'Tweet' and went back to seeing my patients. When I checked my phone a few hours later there had been a modest, but extremely positive response. Those who had read the thread seemed genuinely moved, and were sharing it with their friends on other social media platforms. Some slightly higher profile accounts (like the inimitable and lovely Gus Silber) retweeted the thread and I was pleased that people were getting meaning from it. It was during dinner that I realised the tweets had taken off. Influential accounts with huge followings were commenting and retweeting, and the thread had gone international. The number of retweets and likes were increasing so exponentially that my phone couldn't keep up. When I went to bed the thread had 19 000 likes. When I woke up it was 45 000 and news agencies and television outlets were reaching out.

Going 'viral' is a strange experience. In your Twitter bubble, things are exploding and it's all very exciting. Meanwhile, in the outside world, most people who either aren't on Twitter, or use it very sparingly, couldn't care less and have no idea. You're both famous and unknown at the same time.

So many bereaved parents who had lost children reached out to express their gratitude for the thread, which brought back fond memories of what made the relationship with their children so meaningful. Many others thought that it provided them with direction and clarity. One children's author wrote, 'You mean ... the work I do provides joy to kids in pain? It lessens suffering and provides joy? Well THAT CHANGES EVERYTHING! I was close to suicide, but how could I end things when I have such important work to do. Time to get writing!'

Many said they were putting down their pens, laptops and cellphones and taking their kids for ice cream.

I ended up doing interviews with BBC, Sky and a host of other radio stations and news outlets. I honestly remember very little of what I said, except to reiterate that there was nothing fundamentally new or profound about what I had tweeted. Most people already know that what matters isn't money, or fame, or power. Plenty of people with all three are completely miserable. Rather, it's family, fun, pets and quality time that count. But the world has become such a confusing and opaque place that having these important messages reiterated by the most innocent really resonated. People are hungry for guidance and meaning and these kids, in their unassuming way, offered it.

As with all things in life, whenever there is praise and enjoyment for something, there are contrarians to explain how what we like is awful. I was accused of exploiting dying children for clicks and fame (even though I had explicitly asked their permission to share what they told me). I was told I was profiting off suffering and cynically milking pain for superficial aphorisms. The criticisms stung and I tried my best to avoid them. I took the good advice of 'Don't read the comment section' whenever I was featured in a news article.

And suddenly … it was over. The phrase 'Five minutes of fame' is truly apt. One moment I was the flavour of Twitter, and a few days later people had moved on. The thread ultimately garnered over twenty million views, nearly a 100 000 likes and retweets, and is still there, albeit in a broken state (the sheer volume of responses broke the app's ability to cope). Many of the people who started following me drifted away when they realised my account was primarily focused on debunking medical misinformation and promoting vaccines and heavy metal bands, instead of ongoing blueprints about how to live. That wisdom came from the children, not me. I cannot claim to be an expert on how to find happiness except to say: we should listen to the kids (and eat more ice cream).

A few months later, a hospital in Canada offered me a fellowship position in paediatric infectious diseases. I had realised, over time, that while palliative care had forever changed me, it was not something I could sustain for the entirety of my career. Neither my heart nor my soul could handle the nature of the work forever. My work at PaedsPal had been a placeholder while waiting for a position in Cape Town. Despite my best efforts, that post never materialised, and when I was offered the opportunity to study abroad, I took it. I had always wanted to spend some time overseas, and with a collapsing marriage and a stagnant career, this seemed as good a time as any. I hope, one day soon, to return to the complicated country I love.

My life as a paediatrician goes on, forever altered by my experiences with addiction, my crazy time at Baragwanath, and my experiences with children requiring palliative care.

I still listen to metal music every day, and it still provides me with the peace and joy it did when I was finding myself. *Sunbather* remains my favourite album, although my tastes have broadened considerably. Almost everyone I meet remains totally bemused about my taste in music, but I don't care. I found the music that moves me. I hope you find the music that moves you (if you haven't, I have a few recommendations ...).

I hope this memoir convinces people that medicine is still a worthwhile career choice, that addiction is not a moral failing, and that we should be more honest with how we deal with it in the medical field. Substance abuse is sadly pervasive among physicians, many of whom use it as a strategy to cope with the pain they see every day. It ranges from drinking a little too much at the end of a long day, to stealing fentanyl from anaesthetic trolleys. It isn't spoken about because once you have the label of an 'impaired physician' stamped like a mark of shame on your record, it can follow you around for the rest of your career. Many choose, instead, to stay silent; some take their own lives. The tides are changing, and

PRESCRIPTION: ICE CREAM

many healthcare workers are opening up about their mental-health issues, but we have a long way to go. To anyone reading this who is struggling, please know that help is out there, recovery is possible, and I hope you reach out. Find a professional or someone else who achieved sobriety and do what they tell you to. The cycle of misery *can* be broken.

I don't know the key to happiness, but I do know that it isn't found at the bottom of a bottle or the end of a syringe. You may just find it, however, sitting quietly with a child, eating your favourite ice cream.

Acknowledgements

Writing this book has been one of the most rewarding yet challenging experiences of my life. It would not have been possible without the guidance and support of so many.

To Laura, my beautiful partner, who gave me the space and encouragement to write, even when we had a newborn at home, and I should have been doing laundry instead. You soften me when the world threatens to make me hard and cold.

To my parents, Roy and Helen, who never gave up on me, even when I had given up on myself. Thank you for always seeing the best version of me.

To my siblings, David and Claire, who always felt I had a story to tell, even when I wasn't sure anyone would care.

To my colleagues in palliative care and PaedsPal: you show us the very best humanity has to offer. I am so grateful you let me work with you.

To the people in recovery, who could stay home, but instead go to empty halls and churches to show others how to find another way: thank you.

I would not have finished *Prescription: Ice Cream* without my 'wise owl' and publisher, Andrea Nattrass, who provided support when

I was full of doubt, patience when I was overwhelmed, and advice when I was stuck. Thank you. And thank you for kicking my bum when it needed kicking.

I am also indebted to the encouragement and superb editorial skills of Jane Bowman, and the entire communications team at Pan Macmillan, without whom the story you have read would still be fragments floating in my brain.

Finally, I am inspired every day by the wisdom and courage of the children I treat. In particular, by those forced to confront their own mortality far too soon. I will never know why you chose such an imperfect vessel for your message, but I am forever honoured.